# The ECG Workbook

Angela Rowlands

Andrew Sargent

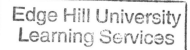
**The ECG Workbook 2nd edition**
Angela Rowlands and Andrew Sargent

ISBN: 978-1-905539-77-2

First published 2008
Revised edition published 2011
All illustrations © Andrew Sargent 2007

**British Library Cataloguing in Publication Data**
A catalogue record for this book is available from the British Library

**Notice**
Clinical practice and medical knowledge constantly evolve. Standard safety precautions must be followed,
but, as knowledge is broadened by research, changes in practice, treatment and drug therapy may become
necessary or appropriate. Readers must check the most current product information provided by the manufacturer of each drug to be administered and verify the dosages and correct administration, as well as con-
traindications. It is the responsibility of the practitioner, utilising the experience and knowledge of the patient,
to determine dosages and the best treatment for each individual patient. Any brands mentioned in this book
are as examples only and are not endorsed by the Publisher. Neither the Publisher nor the authors assume
any liability for any injury and/or damage to persons or property arising from this publication.

*The Publisher*

To contact M&K Publishing write to:
M&K Update Ltd · The Old Bakery · St. Johns Street
Keswick · Cumbria CA12 5AS
Tel: 01768 773030 · Fax: 01768 781099
publishing@mkupdate.co.uk
www.mkupdate.co.uk

Designed and typeset in 11pt Usherwood Book by Mary Blood
Printed in England by Reeds Limited, Penrith

# Contents

## Preface to the second edition

When we made our first faltering steps as nurses in coronary care, we were in awe of the gifted band of nurses and doctors who discussed the mysteries of electrocardiograms (ECGs) in what seemed like an alien tongue. It was only after we were given an explanation in plain English that ECG interpretation started to make sense and we were able to relate the ECG to the patient.

This book takes a straightforward, systematic approach to ECG interpretation. We have tried to present the subject in an easily digestible form to those setting out in this discipline, without burdening our readers with unnecessary jargon.

Each step in the process of recording and interpreting an ECG is presented in sequence, in its own chapter. At the end of each chapter there are a number of activities to help readers practise what they have learned, evaluate their learning and relate their learning to patient scenarios. Answers are provided at the back of the book.

You will find a number of words in bold text throughout the book. These are words that may be new to you if you have a limited experience in Cardiology. A full explanation of the meaning of these terms can be found in the glossary at the back of the book.

We have found that many books on ECG interpretation use simulated ECG tracings. Most of the tracings that you find in this book are from real people and of the quality that you will be expected to interpret from in practice.

Following the publication of the first edition of *The ECG Workbook*, we were pleased with the positive response we received from reviewers and clinicians. The popularity of the book seemed to be largely due to the systematic approach that we had taken in mastering this complex skill. Whilst we were happy with the original book, we felt that there was scope to develop it further.

There are two new chapters in this second edition that we feel add greatly to the usefulness of the book. Firstly, there is now a chapter on 'Common arrhythmias'. Throughout the book, there are numerous references to arrhythmias that you are likely to encounter in practice, but we felt that there should be a dedicated chapter to help you understand and recognise them. Secondly, we have included a chapter on 'Ectopics and extrasystoles', as we recognise that these frequently appear on ECGs but their significance is often misunderstood.

Both these new chapters adhere to the principles we followed when we started work on the first edition: that the text should be accessible and relevant to all practitoners, regardless of their experience, and that the text should always be supported with relevant exercises to reinforce learning.

*Andrew Sargent and Angela Rowlands, March 2011*

## About the authors

**Angela Rowlands** is currently a Lecturer at St Barts and the Royal London Medical School, Queen Mary University of London. Angela is a qualified nurse with over 20 years of clinical experience in Cardiology. She is a qualified teacher and for many years combined her clinical work with education in the roles of Practice Educator for Cardiology and as Senior Lecturer at Thames Valley University, Berkshire where she set up and ran the Coronary Care Nursing course. She lives in Oxfordshire with her husband John and two children Thomas and Ben.

**Andrew Sargent** is a Tutor in Critical Care Nursing at the Florence Nightingale School of Nursing and Midwifery, King's College London. Andrew has extensive experience as an educator and has a clinical background in Cardiology and Cardiac ICU. He lives in London with his wife Zoe and two children Lara and Alex.

## Dedication

Angela – In memory of my mother Janet Rees, 1942–2007
Andrew – For Zoe, Lara and Alex and to my mother and father for all their love and support

# Chapter 1

# *Recording a readable electrocardiogram (ECG)*

An ECG is a graphic tracing of electrical patterns produced by the heart. This test is frequently used for patients who have heart problems and is an important diagnostic procedure. However, the ECG has limitations and so it is important to evaluate it in conjunction with the patient's clinical status. ECG abnormalities can occur in healthy individuals; and it can also be possible for a person to have a heart attack and yet have a normal ECG. The nature of the abnormality and its effect on the patient influence the clinical importance of the findings, so the ECG should never be used in isolation.

Before we start to interpret the ECG, it is important to learn how to obtain a readable recording (see fig 1.1). We will learn in the following chapters that slight changes can have huge implications for the patient. These days it is common for ancillary staff to take on the task of recording ECGs. To the untrained eye a recording may seem readable but it is not until we learn to interpret an ECG recording that we really gain an understanding of the importance of producing a readable tracing. It is possible to misdiagnose patients or miss their diagnosis if the recording is not clear.

Before interpreting the ECG, it is therefore essential to ensure that the recording was obtained correctly. Common errors are incorrect paper speed and standardisation, **artefact** and incorrect lead placement. Any of these problems can make it extremely difficult, and in some cases impossible, to measure the intervals and the segments that we are going to learn about in this book.

## Paper speed and standardisation

The ECG is made up of a series of horizontal and vertical lines that measure the duration and amplitude of the various deflections. The small boxes on the paper are 1 millimetre (mm) in height and I mm in width. The amplitude of the ECG deflection is measured vertically and the duration of the ECG event horizontally. Recordings are usually made at 25 mm per second (mm/s). It is therefore important to ensure that the ECG machine has not been set, at say, 50mm/s before the ECG is recorded. The paper speed should be printed on the ECG itself when it is recorded (see fig 1.2).

A standard deflection (a box that looks like half a rectangle) should be inscribed at the beginning or end of the ECG. The ECG is usually standardised so that the amplitude of a 1 millivolt impulse causes a deflection of 10 mm (see fig 1.3). An increased amplitude (or voltage) usually indicates increased muscle mass of the heart.

*Note: If the ECG is not set at 25 mm/s, all the usual ECG measurements that we are about to learn will not apply.*

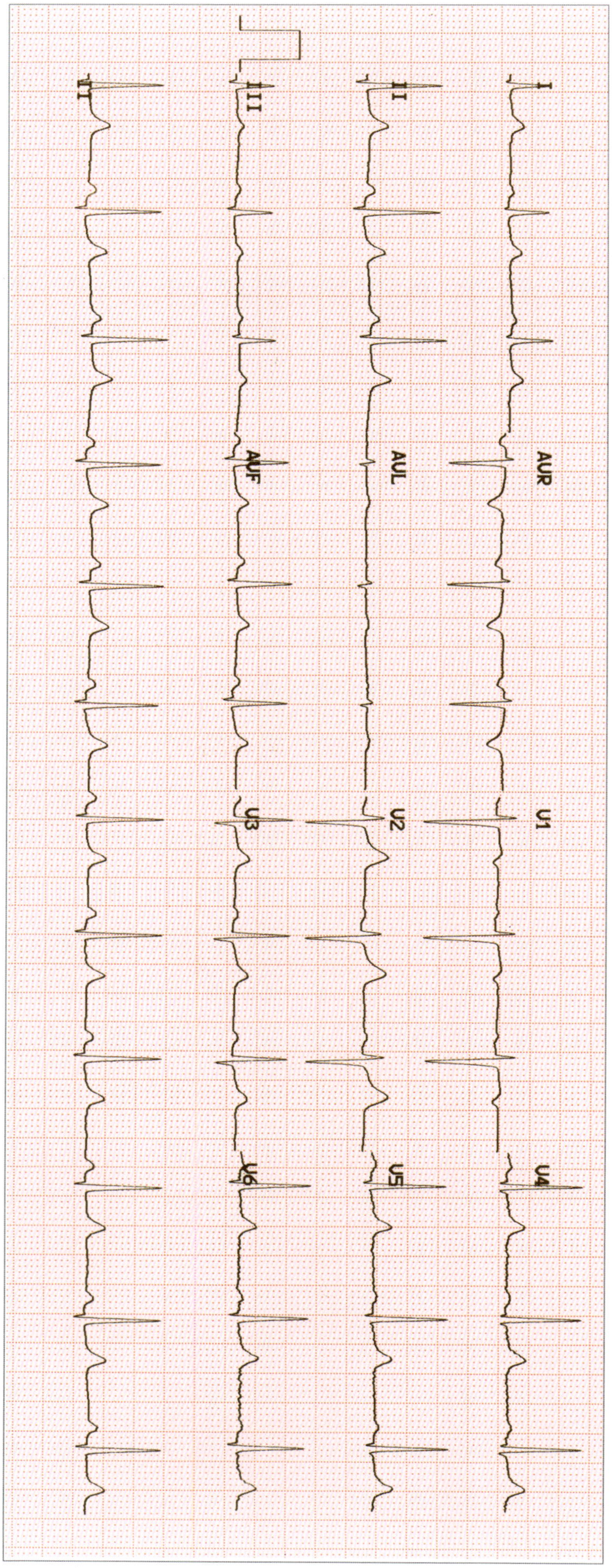

**Figure 1.1:** *A 12 lead ECG with many normal features*

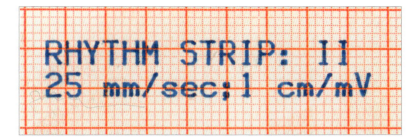

**Figure 1.2:** *The paper (or 'sweep') speed printed on an ECG.*

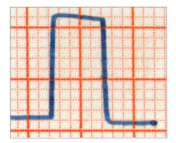

**Figure 1.3:** *The standard deflection at the end of an ECG.*

## Artefact

To obtain a good-quality ECG tracing you need to make sure that there is no outside interference, as this can create artefact. The three most common causes of artefact are:

1  mains interference

2  patient movement

3  wandering baseline.

### Mains interference

Mains interference may produce a fuzzy trace. Too much or too little heat stimulus will produce a tracing that is too thick or too faint. Mains interference usually comes from electrical interaction at or near the patient's bedside. For this reason, any pumps or electric fans situated nearby should be switched off or left to run on battery while the ECG is being recorded. Interference can also occur if the patient is in contact with metal, such as the end of the bed, or if an ECG lead is in contact with metal (e.g. touching a watch) or the ECG leads are tangled. Recording the ECG with the machine on battery status instead of mains also helps to eliminate mains interference.

### Patient movement

If the patient is tense or moving during the recording, artefact will result. What may be a routine procedure to a healthcare professional is not always a routine procedure to a patient. Learning that the healthcare professional wants to take a tracing of their heart is not exactly conducive to relaxation! For instance, patients have been known to express concern that they might get electrocuted if the healthcare professional gets the leads in the wrong order! For all these reasons it is important to explain to the patient the aim of the procedure, that it will not hurt, that it will only take a few minutes and that it will help if they can relax as much as possible, as this will produce a clearer recording. It is often helpful to ask patients to close their eyes and imagine themselves somewhere relaxing.

Many patients feel embarrassed about having their chests exposed for an ECG recording. Always ensure their privacy during the recording. Remember also that some patients may concentrate on your facial expression in an attempt to assess your reaction to the ECG as it is being printed. You should therefore try to keep your expression as neutral as possible.

### Wandering baseline

Wandering baseline makes it difficult to identify ECG changes, as many of these changes are measured from the baseline. This problem is often caused by poor electrode contact with the skin. You might need to ask permission to shave some of the hair off the patient's chest in order to obtain good electrode contact. It may also be necessary to dry the skin if the patient is sweating, or clean the skin if talcum powder has been applied. Ensure that the skin is completely dry after cleaning.

## Lead placement

ECG electrodes must be placed in the correct positions on the body. If they are not, changes could appear on the recording that are simply caused by looking at the heart from a slightly different angle. This could easily lead to misdiagnosis. It would also make comparison of the patient's ECG recordings unreliable.

The limb leads are labelled: R (right), L (left), F (foot) and N (neutral). The R lead should be attached to the patient's inner, right wrist; the L lead to the inner, left wrist; the F lead to the inner left leg (just above the ankle); and the N lead in the same position on the right leg (see fig 1.4).

Ideally electrodes should be placed over fleshy surfaces, as flesh conducts electricity much better than bone. It is important to have the leads the right way round, otherwise this could change the **polarity** of the **ECG complexes**. What is being measured from these leads is simply the difference in electrical potential between two points, so if these points vary slightly (e.g. in a patient with an amputation), one would simply attach the leads higher up the leg.

It is vital, however, to get the position of the chest electrodes correct (see fig 1.5):

1 V1 should be positioned in the fourth **intercostal** space counting down from the patient's right sternal notch on the right sternal edge;
2 V2 should be positioned in the fourth intercostal space counting down from the patient's left **sternal notch on the left sternal edge**;
3 V3 should be positioned midway between V2 and V4;
4 V4 should be positioned in the fifth intercostal space, counting down from the middle of the patient's **clavicle**;
5 V5 should be positioned in line with V4 but on the **anterior axillary line**;
6 V6 should be positioned in line with V4 but in the **midaxillary line**.

The position of the patient will also make a difference to the ECG recording, as different positions alter the way the heart lies within the chest wall. The ECG should be recorded with the patient lying flat, with two pillows under their head. Some patients (e.g. patients with acute breathlessness) will not tolerate lying flat. In such cases it should be noted on the ECG that the patient was not lying flat, so that the interpreter can take this into account when analysing the ECG. Before the leads are disconnected, the quality of the ECG should be examined. If there is any distortion of the trace, the source of the distortion must be identified and corrected, and the ECG must then be carried out again.

It is essential to record the patient's name and the date and time of the recording on the ECG. The interpreter of the ECG will also find it useful to know whether the patient was experiencing any symptoms at the time of the recording.

Remember to leave the ECG machine clean, untangled and ready for use at all times, as it is often needed in emergency situations.

Chapter 1, Activity 1 (page 6) describes the process of recording a cardiac rhythm strip for analysis.

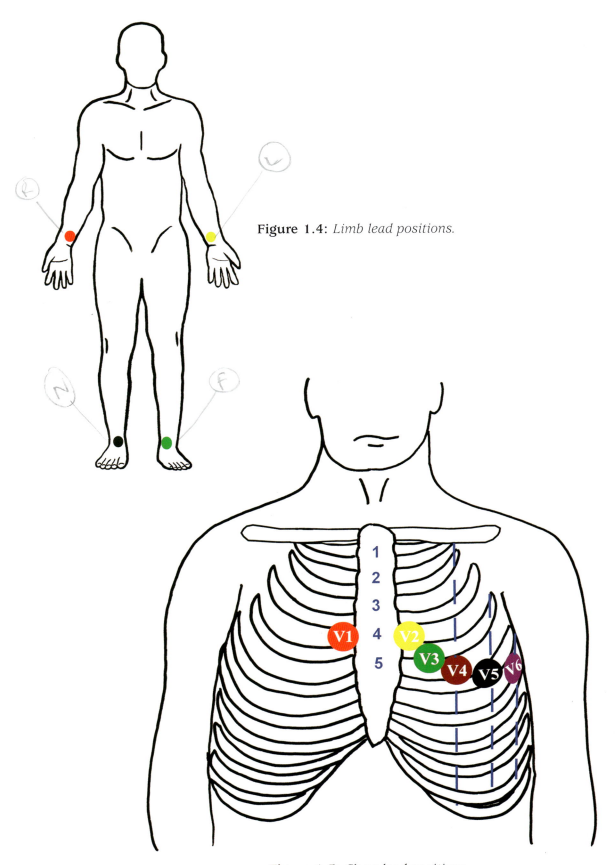

**Figure 1.4:** *Limb lead positions.*

**Figure 1.5:** *Chest lead positions.*

# Chapter 1 activity

Chapter 1 explains how to carry out an accurate recording of a 12 lead ECG.

Make sure that you have read through the chapter and that you have fully understood the key concepts presented. Then work through the following activity.

Once you have completed this activity, you should be able to:

- place leads in the correct position for a 12 lead ECG recording;
- record a clear, accurate 12 lead ECG.

### Activity 1.1: Recording a 12 lead ECG

*Approximate time needed to complete this exercise:* 10 minutes
*What you will need:*

- a 12 lead ECG recorder;
- ECG electrodes;
- a subject (a patient or colleague) who has about 10 minutes to spare.

1  Ask your subject to lie down as flat as possible. Tell them to relax and rest their arms at their sides and to loosen any items of clothing that are tight or may cause them discomfort.
2  Remove clothing from the patient's upper body as necessary in order to expose the chest. Any items of clothing that will obstruct the application of the chest electrodes should be moved or removed. Remember to protect the subject's dignity and privacy at all times.
3  Identify the important anatomical landmarks required for lead positioning (see fig 1.4 and 1.5 on p. 4 if you need to remind yourself of where these are).
4  Identify any potential problems with the lead placement. For example, do any clothes or underwear need to be removed?
5  Assess the skin areas where the leads will be placed. Is the skin clean and dry? Is the skin excessively hairy? Identify the measures required to ensure that the electrodes will make good contact with the skin.
6  Place the leads on the limbs and the chest in accordance with the diagrams in fig 1.4 and 1.5 (p. 5).
7  Record the ECG in accordance with the manufacturer's instructions for your ECG recorder.
8  Examine your ECG for the following:
   - the paper ("sweep") speed should be printed on the ECG paper (see fig 1.2, p. 2);
   - the electrical calibration signal should be printed – this is often shown at the end of each printed rhythm on the paper (see fig 1.3, p. 3);
   - check for signs of interference or wandering baseline;
   - check that each section of the 12 lead ECG has recorded properly and that there is not a straight line.
9  If you are happy that your ECG has recorded properly, remove the electrodes and thank your subject for their cooperation.

You should now have a well-recorded 12 lead ECG. Don't worry if you don't understand what all these ECG complexes mean at the moment. Keep this recording and use it for later activities in this book. Soon it will all make sense!

## Chapter 2

# The electrical conducting system of the heart

The heart has specialised cells that form its conducting system. Electrical impulses are initiated and conducted from within the heart. These impulses produce myocardial contraction. It is these electrical impulses that are recorded on cardiac monitors and the electrocardiogram.

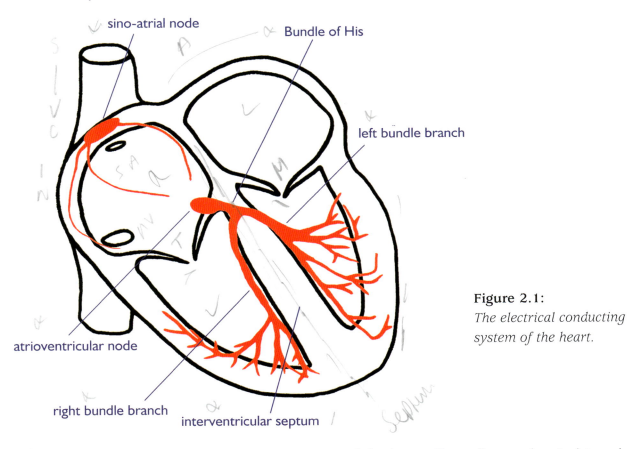

**Figure 2.1:**
*The electrical conducting system of the heart.*

Figure 2.1 shows the electrical conducting system of the heart. Normally, an electrical impulse comes from the sino-atrial (SA) node, which is situated in the right **atrium** close to the entrance of the **vena cava**. The impulse then spreads across the atria to the atrioventricular node (AV), which lies in the right atrial wall above the **tricuspid valve**. It then reaches the **ventricles** by passing through the Bundle of His and into the bundle branches. The left and right bundle branches, which extend along the interventricular **septum**, conduct the impulse to the ventricular **myocardium** to cause it to contract. The first part of the ventricles to be activated is the septum, followed by the **endocardium** and then the **epicardium**.

The ECG records the movement of these electrical impulses and the wave pattern generated is known as the **PQRST complex**.

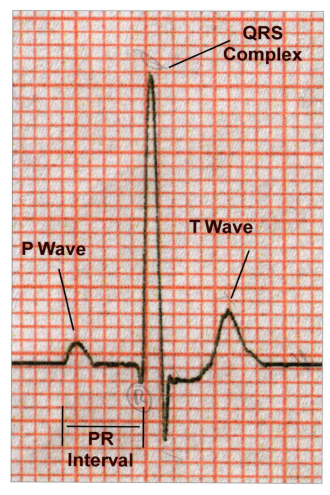

**Figure 2.2:** *The PQRST complex.*

1 The *P wave* represents the spread of the impulse from the SA node across the atria (often referred to as atrial **depolarisation**).

2 The *PR interval* represents the time taken for the impulse to spread over the atrium and through the AV node, where the impulse pauses for a short time.

3 The *QRS complex* represents the spread of the impulse through the ventricles (ventricular depolarisation).

4 The *T wave* represents ventricular recovery (often referred to as **repolarisation**).

If an impulse travels through the conducting system, being initiated from the SA node in the manner described above, the rhythm is described as a *sinus rhythm*.

# Chapter 2 activities

Chapter 2 has introduced you to the ECG complex and you are now beginning to see how the electrical conducting system is represented on the ECG.

When you have completed the two activities below, you should be able to:

● describe the main components of the electrical conducting system of the heart;

● recognise the elements of the ECG complex and relate them to the relevant part of the conducting system;

● identify the PQRST on a rhythm strip.

### Activity 2.1: Describe the electrical conducting system and the ECG

*Approximate time needed to complete this exercise: 5 minutes*
*Answers are provided on p. 87.*

Fill the gaps in the following passage using the terms you have learned in Chapter 2.

The ECG records electrical __impulse__ as they pass through the __SA__ cells of the _____ system. As the electrical impulses pass across these cells, myocardial _____ occurs. Normally, all electrical impulses originate from the _____ node in the _____ _____. After spreading across the _____, the impulses then pass through the _____ _____ and into the _____ __ _____. The impulse spreads through the _____ _____ via the right and left _____ _____.

Finally, the impulse conducts across the _____ _____, causing contraction.

The ECG is made up of a number of parts, each of which relates to a different part of the conducting system. The first part of the normal ECG complex is the ___ wave. This represents the impulses that arise from the _____ _____ and spread across the _____ towards the _____ node. As the impulse spreads across the ventricular myocardium, the ECG records a large wave called the _____ _____. The spread of impulse across the atria and ventricles is often referred to as _____.

The total time that it takes for depolarisation to spread from the SA node to the ventricular myocardium is measured on the ECG as the ____ _____. When the ventricles recover from depolarisation, the final part of the ECG complex is recorded. This is the _____ _____ and represents _____ of the ventricles.

**Activities 2**

### Activity 2.2: Recognising the parts of an ECG

*Approximate time needed to complete this exercise: 2 minutes*

Look at the rhythm strip on the 12 lead ECG that you recorded in the activity for Chapter 1 (p. 6).

In your head, identify each of the following parts and then label them on the ECG:

1  the P wave

2  the PR interval

3  the QRS complex

4  the T wave.

If you don't see every part of the ECG and it doesn't look like the one in Figure 2.2, don't worry! It may be perfectly normal. As you develop your ECG analysis skills you will start to recognise normal variations in ECG complexes as well as learning about the abnormalities that can be seen.

*You may find it helpful to refer back to Chapters 1 and 2 when you are attempting these two activities, but see how much you can do on your own first.*

# Chapter 3

# A systematic approach to rhythm strip analysis

Figure 3.1 shows a normal 12 lead ECG. The first step in our systematic approach to analysing a 12 lead ECG is to examine the rhythm strip. This is the strip at the bottom of the ECG, which tells us if the electrical impulses are travelling through the conducting system in the correct manner. You will see from the rhythm strip in Figure 3.1 that there are many PQRST complexes linked together. However, there is more information to be gathered from the rhythm strip.

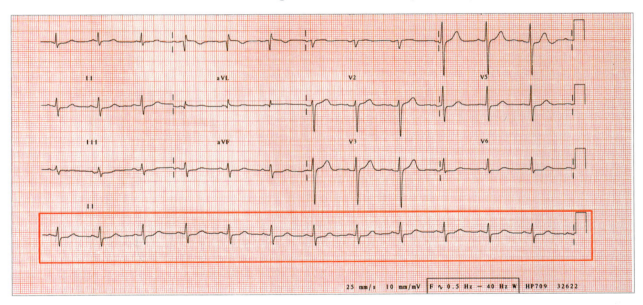

**Figure 3.1:**
*A normal 12 lead ECG reading. Note that the rhythm strip appears along the bottom (in the red box).*

## How can you calculate a patient's heart rate?

When patients are attached to cardiac monitors, a heart rate numerical counter will display how fast their heart is beating. However, this reading can sometimes be inaccurate. For example, if the patient is moving or touching the chest electrodes, the rate counter may pick up the artefact and count this as well as the patient's QRS complexes. Sometimes patients will have small *ectopic* (or extra) beats. These can be very small and may not be picked up by the rate counter, which could once again give an inaccurate reading. We therefore need a reliable way of calculating heart rates from rhythm strips to avoid the danger of a patient being given a drug to alter their heart rate when it is not needed.

One of the easiest ways to calculate heart rate from an ECG strip is firstly to calculate 6 seconds worth of rhythm strip (this equals 30 of the big squares on the ECG graph paper). Then count the number of QRS complexes that fall within these 30 big squares. Multiply this number by 10. This calculation will give you the number of beats per minute (see fig 3.2) and this method works for irregular as well as regular rhythms.

- The normal ventricular heart rate at rest is 60–100 beats per minute.

- A heart rate below 60 beats per minute is termed a bradycardia.

- A heart rate above 100 beats per minute is a tachycardia.

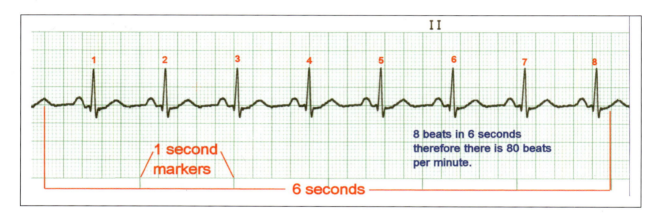

**Figure 3.2:** *A simple method of calculating the heart rate from a rhythm strip. An ECG will normally have 1-second (5 large squares) or 3-second markers (15 large squares).*

### Is the heartbeat rhythm regular or irregular?

Normally, the heart beats in a regular manner. In some rhythm strips it is easy to see if the rhythm is regular because the distances between the QRS complexes look the same. However, problems sometimes arise in faster heart rates, when the beat-to-beat variation of irregular rhythms seems less clear.

One simple way to check whether the rhythm is regular or irregular is to mark the positions of the tips of two or three adjacent QRS complexes on a piece of paper. You can then slide this pattern along the top of the rhythm strip. If the marks align, the rhythm is regular.

### Is there atrial activity?

The next step is to check whether atrial activity is present on the rhythm strip. We have already learned that atrial activity is represented by the presence of a P wave.

### Is there ventricular activity? If so, is it broad, narrow or normal?

Now you need to confirm the presence of ventricular activity on the rhythm strip. We have already learned that ventricular activity is represented by the presence of a QRS complex.

We will learn later on in this chapter that there is a normal time value for each part of the PQRST complex. We can measure these time intervals using the squares on the ECG graph paper. **The upper limit for the width of the QRS complex is 0.12 seconds** (or 3 small squares). If the QRS width is less than 0.12 seconds, the rhythm originates from the atria. If the QRS duration is more than 0.12 seconds, the rhythm may be arising from the ventricles. This can be dangerous for the patient, as the ventricles are responsible for pumping the blood around the body.

> **REMEMBER:**
> - If the QRS is narrow or normal, the rhythm is usually atrial in origin.
> - If the QRS is broad, the rhythm is usually ventricular in origin.

### What is the relationship between the atrial activity and the ventricular activity?

The next step is to look at the rhythm strip and assess whether there is a normal relationship between the atrial activity and the ventricular activity.

If there is a normal relationship, **there is one P wave before each QRS complex.**

> **REMEMBER:**
> If the relationship between the atrial activity and the ventricular activity is not normal, it may be a heart block (see Chapter 4, pp. 19–23).

### Measuring the intervals

At this point you need to look at all the waves previously mentioned to assess whether they fit their precisely defined time intervals. You can do this by looking at the ECG graph paper. Figure 3.3 (below) shows that the big squares, and the small squares within them, have certain time values:

**1 small square = 0.04 seconds**

**1 big square = 0.20 seconds**

There are 5 small squares in each big square so:
0.04 seconds x 5 = 0.20 seconds.

### The P wave

You should start by measuring the duration of the P wave, from where the P wave starts to where it ends. This should not exceed 0.08 seconds in duration. A patient may have an abnormally wide P wave, for example, when there is left atrial hypertrophy (see Chapter 12, p. 81). In this case the impulse would take longer to travel through the large atrial wall and so the P wave would be wider than normal and often notched like a letter m.

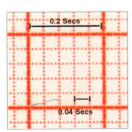

**Figure 3.3:** *Time values on ECG graph paper.*

### The PR interval

The next step is to measure the PR interval. This represents the time taken for atrial depolarisation and AV node delay. It is measured from the start of the P wave to the beginning of the QRS complex and is normally 0.12–0.20 seconds in duration. The PR interval lengthens if the impulse pauses for too long in the AV node (this is called AV block or **heart block** and will be dealt with in Chapter 4). A shortened PR interval is seen when the impulse originates in the tissues of the AV node or if a person has a congenital abnormality (such as Wolff–Parkinson–White syndrome), where there is an accessory pathway that bypasses the AV node.

## The QRS complex

The QRS complex is measured from when the deflection first leaves the baseline (either in a positive or negative deflection), after the PR interval, to when it returns to the baseline just before the T wave. As previously mentioned, a value of greater than 0.12 seconds is abnormal and usually indicates a conduction disorder within the ventricles.

## QT interval

The QT interval represents the total time from the onset of ventricular depolarisation to repolarisation. It is measured from the beginning of the QRS complex to the end of the T wave. Its duration varies with heart rate: it gets shorter as heart rate increases. The relationship between heart rate and QT intervals is a complex one; and some ECG books include tables that calculate QT intervals according to heart rate.

Essentially, the QT interval should be less than 50 per cent of the preceding cycle length. In practice, you can analyse most rhythm strips using the above systematic approach and reach a diagnosis without being able to work out the QT interval. However, a prolonged QT interval has been associated with a risk of ventricular tachycardia and torsades de pointes (rhythms of cardiac arrest). It has also been linked with congenital abnormalities and the use of some drugs (such as amioderone and tricyclic anti-depressants).

> **REMEMBER:**
> P wave = < 0.08 seconds
> PR interval = 0.12–0.20 seconds
> QRS complex = < 0.12 seconds

## Naming or describing an ECG

When you first start learning how to interpret ECGs you may be put off by the complicated names of cardiac rhythm abnormalities (known as arrhythmias). It is not necessary to learn all the rhythm names at this stage. What is important is to be able to identify abnormalities and know how these abnormalities may affect a patient.

> **REMEMBER:**
> Precise ECG classification is by no means vital. It's far more important to recognise how the abnormal rhythm is compromising the patient's cardiac output and obtain appropriate treatment for the patient. The same arrhythmia often has different consequences for different patients.

After assessing your patient, if you cannot name the rhythm, simply describe the abnormalities over the telephone to a colleague who understands cardiology. Your colleague will then be able to identify the rhythm abnormality and administer appropriate emergency treatment if required.

Figure 3.4 (below) shows a rhythm abnormality. Applying the systematic approach described above, it can be analysed as follows:

*Rate* = 220 beats per minute (bpm)

*Rhythm* = regular

*Atrial activity* = no P waves

*Ventricular activity* = present and broad

*Relationship* = unable to comment as no visible P waves

*Intervals:*
- P wave = none
- PR interval = none
- QRS = 0.28 secs

*Description:* A broad complex tachycardia of 220bpm.

The name of this rhythm is **ventricular tachycardia.**

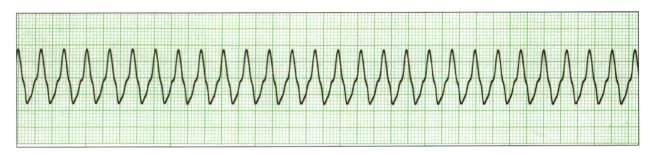

**Figure 3.4:** *Ventricular tachycardia.*

## SUMMARY: Rhythm strip analysis

- Rate?
- Rhythm? Regular or irregular?
- Atrial activity?
- Ventricular activity? Broad, narrow or normal?
- Relationship?
- Intervals?
- Name/description?

**Activities 3**

# Chapter 3 activities

You are now well on your way to performing a full analysis of an ECG using a systematic analysis tool. The following activities will enable you to practise these skills further so that you become more familiar with the tool and the ECG as a whole.

The activities present two case scenarios with their accompanying ECG rhythm strips, and you should use the analysis tool to identify the abnormality in each case. At this stage you are not expected to name the arrhythmia in question or to describe how it has come about. (Those aspects will be covered in later chapters.) The important goal here is to recognise the normal and abnormal features.

When you have completed the two activities below, you should be able to:

● recognise abnormal features of an ECG complex;

● begin to put the abnormal rhythm strip in the context of a patient scenario.

### Activity 3.1: Rhythm strip analysis

*Approximate time required to complete this exercise: 10 minutes*
*Answers are provided on p. 87.*

### Scenario 1

Mrs Smith is a 68-year-old lady who has a recent history of feeling short of breath on minimal exertion. She has also been feeling fatigued and occasionally light headed. She has had the following ECG recorded at her GP's surgery.

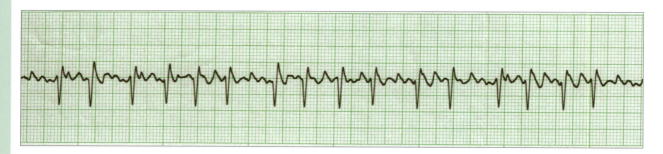

**Figure 3.5:** *Mrs Smith's ECG.*

Using your analysis tool, complete the following table:

| What is the rate? | |
|---|---|
| Is it regular or irregular? | |
| Is there atrial activity? (P waves) | |
| Is there ventricular activity? (QRS complexes) | |
| Are the QRS complexes broad or narrow? | |
| Is there a relationship between the atrial activity and the ventricular activity? | |
| Are the PR intervals normal? | |
| Name/description? | |

**Scenario 2**

Mr Jones is a 46-year-old man who has been suffering with a chest infection for several days and is being treated with oral antibiotics. His oral temperature is 37.5°C. Today, he developed chest pain across his left lower thorax. An ECG is taken to exclude a possible cardiac cause of this pain (see fig 3.6).

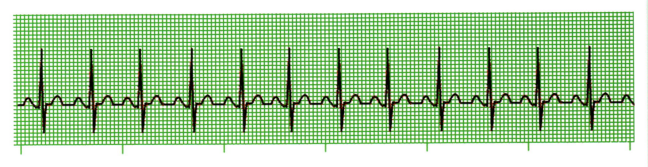

**Figure 3.6:** *Mr Jones's ECG.*

Using your analysis tool, complete the following table:

| | |
|---|---|
| What is the rate? | |
| Is it regular or irregular? | |
| Is there atrial activity? (P waves) | |
| Is there ventricular activity? (QRS complexes) | |
| Are the QRS complexes broad or narrow? | |
| Is there a relationship between the atrial activity and the ventricular activity? | |
| Are the PR intervals normal? | |
| Name/description? | |

## Activity 3.2: More rhythm strip interpretation

*Approximate time required to complete this activity: 10 minutes*

Use the rhythm strip on the 12 lead ECG that you recorded in Chapter 1 (see p. 6) to perform further analyses, using the same tool. Record any abnormalities in the table below.

| | Analysis |
|---|---|
| What is the rate? | |
| Is it regular or irregular? | |
| Is there atrial activity? (P waves) | |
| Is there ventricular activity? (QRS complexes) | |
| Are the QRS complexes broad or narrow? | |
| Is there a relationship between the atrial activity and the ventricular activity? | |
| Are the PR intervals normal? | |

**NB:** It would be a good idea to start collecting a few ECGs for your own use. You can either take recordings from your colleagues, or you could take some copies of ECGs that you record in your daily practice. Remember to seek permission from the person you are taking the ECG from, and make sure that any personal identifying data is removed in order to protect patient confidentiality.

Chapter 4

# Heart blocks

We learned in the previous chapter that if the relationship between the atrial and ventricular activity is not normal, we may be dealing with a heart block.

Heart blocks (or AV blocks) occur when conduction from the atria to the ventricles is either blocked or slowed. These arrhythmias may be classed as first, second and third degree heart blocks. They may be caused by **fibrosis** of the conducting system, damage from coronary heart disease or as a result of drugs, such as beta blockers or digoxin.

## First degree heart block

First degree heart block is when there is an excessive delay in the electrical impulse being passed through the AV node from the atria to the ventricles. On the ECG this is represented by the prolonged PR interval (see fig 4.1). The prolonged PR interval is always constant.

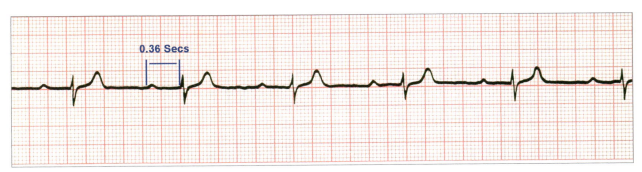

**Figure 4.1:**
*In first degree heart block the PR interval is greater than 0.20 seconds (or one large box on the ECG graph paper).*

## Second degree heart block

There are two types of second degree heart block, Mobitz type I and Mobitz type II.

### Mobitz type I (or the Wenkebach phenomenon)

This is the most common type of second degree heart block. Each successive impulse from the atria finds it more difficult to pass through the AV node. This is represented on the ECG as *the PR interval progressively prolonging with each beat*. Eventually the impulse is unable to pass through to the ventricles and a P wave is not followed by a QRS complex. When the next P wave reaches the AV node it has recovered and conducts normally. Then the pattern repeats. (See Figure 4.2 overpage.)

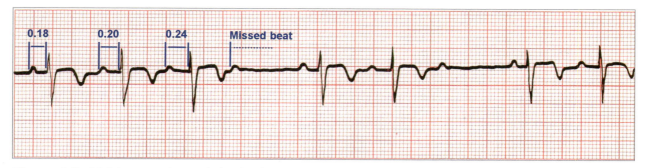

**Figure 4.2:** *Mobitz type I (Wenkebach phenomenon). Note the progressive increase in the duration of the PR interval before a QRS complex is missed. The cycle then begins again.*

### Mobitz type II

Here the AV node randomly fails to respond to some atrial impulses. On the ECG rhythm strip P waves are seen but they are not followed by a QRS complex. When the impulse is passed onto the ventricles the PR intervals are always constant.

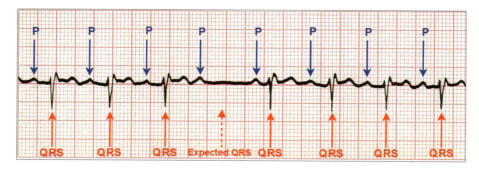

**Figure 4.3:** *Mobitz Type II second degree heart block. Note there is a P wave without a QRS complex however the PR intervals before the QRS complexes are constant.*

In Mobitz Type II the terms 2:1 or 3:1 or varying block are used to describe the number of P waves that are not followed by QRS complexes.

## Third degree (complete) heart block

In third degree heart block there is **no relationship between the P waves and the QRS complexes**. The atria and ventricles are working independently. Atrial impulses can be blocked at the AV node or lower down in the conducting system. If the block is within the AV node the QRS complexes are usually narrow but if the block is within the ventricles the QRS becomes wide.

If the SA node fails, impulses may be initiated from a subsidiary site – located in the atria, at the AV node, or in the ventricles. The resulting rhythm is termed 'an escape rhythm' and will normally be slower than those originating from higher up in the conducting system. In third degree heart block there are two different pacemaker sites, the atria and the ventricles. The site of the pacemaker stimulating the ventricles will determine the ventricle rate (see Figure 4.4 opposite).

## Treatment for heart blocks?

The need for treatment for heart blocks depends on the **haemodynamic** consequences of the arrhythmia, rather than the precise ECG classification of the arrhythmia. First degree heart block produces no symptoms but can deteriorate and lead to the other types of block. If the ventricular rate in second and third degree heart block is sufficiently low (usually below 40 beats per minute), cardiac failure and **hypotension** may be precipitated. Extreme bradycardia may precipitate cardiac arrest so the heart must be accelerated. This may be achieved by inserting an artificial pacemaker.

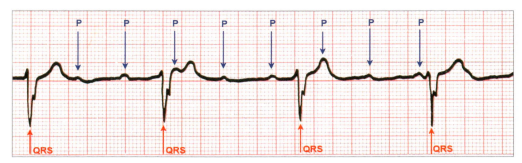

**Figure 4.4:** *Third degree (complete) heart block. Note that there are regular P waves (blue arrows) and there are also regular QRS complexes (red arrows) but there is no relationship between them.*

## SUMMARY: Heart blocks

Is the relationship between the atrial and ventricular activity normal on the ECG strip? If not, could it be a type of heart block? Which pattern does it fit?

| First degree | PR interval > 0.20 seconds |
| --- | --- |
| Second degree<br>● Mobitz type I (Wenkebach)<br>● Mobitz type II | PR gradually gets longer and then drops a beat.<br><br>Dropped beats but PR interval before the QRS complexes are always constant. |
| Third degree | No relationship between atrial and ventricular activity. |

# Chapter 4 activities

Learning to distinguish between the different types of block is very important. It requires a bit of practice at first, as some of the blocks can appear very similar.

In these activities you will look at different types of block, particularly the specific features that differentiate them from each other. You will also be tested on your learning up to this point in the book.

When you have completed the following activities, you should be able to:

● differentiate between first, second and third degree heart block;

● recognise when there is association or dissociation between atrial and ventricular activity;

● understand what you have learned in Chapters 1–4.

Answers are provided on pp. 88–91.

### Activity 4.1: Recognising different AV node blocks
*Approximate time required to complete this activity: 15 minutes*

Look at the following ECG rhythm strips and complete the table below.

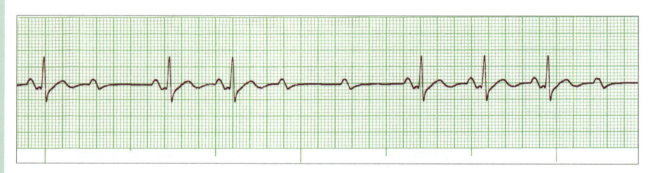

**Figure 4.5:** *ECG 1*

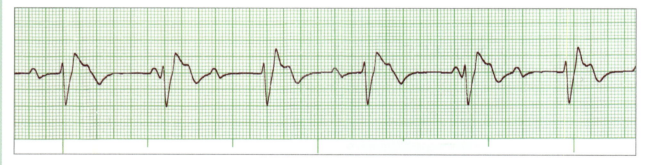

**Figure 4.6:** *ECG 2*

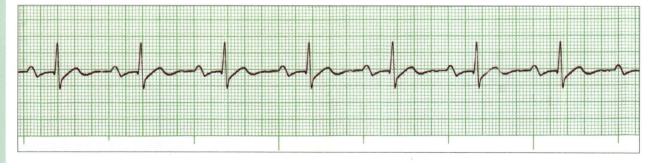

**Figure 4.7:** *ECG 3*

|  | ECG 1 | ECG 2 | ECG 3 |
|---|---|---|---|
| Is there atrial activity? |  |  |  |
| Are the P waves regular? |  |  |  |
| Is the ventricular activity regular? |  |  |  |
| Is the PR interval constant or does it vary? |  |  |  |
| If the PR interval is constant, is it normal? |  |  |  |
| Are there missed QRS complexes? |  |  |  |
| What is this heart block? |  |  |  |

## Activity 4.2: Review of Chapters 1–4

Tick the correct answer.

**1 The ECG represents...**

A The structure of the heart

B Movement of electrical impulses through the heart

C Movement of blood through the heart

D The state of the coronary arteries

**2 Electrical conduction of the heart's cells is also known as...**

A Polarisation

B Repolarisation

C Depolarisation

D Defibrillation

**3 ECG paper speed should be...**

A 25cm/s

B 2.5 mm/s

C 2.5m/s

D 25mm/s

**4 1 millivolt is represented as...**

A 2 large squares on the vertical axis

B 2 cm on the horizontal axis

C 1 large square on the horizontal axis

D 2 cm on the vertical axis

Activities 4

**5 One small square on the horizontal axis of the ECG paper is...**

A  0.4 seconds

B  0.04 seconds

C  1 second

D  0.2 seconds

**6 One large square on the horizontal axis of the ECG paper is...**

A  0.04 seconds

B  1 second

C  0.2 seconds

D  0.02 seconds

**7 Which of these will not cause artefact on an ECG?**

A  Patient movement

B  Electrical apparatus

C  Palpitations

D  Poor electrode contact

**8 Lead V4 is positioned...**

A  In the fourth intercostal space on the right sternal border

B  In the fourth intercostal space on the left sternal border

C  In the fifth intercostal space on the midaxillary line

D  In the fifth intercostal space on the mid-clavicular line

**9 The width of the QRS should be...**

A  < 0.12 seconds

B  > 0.12 seconds

C  0.12–2.0 seconds

D  > 2 seconds

**10 An ECG is 'Sinus' if ...**

A  It has a QRS complex

B  It has a P wave

C  It has a T wave

D  The ventricular rate is regular

**11** Using a pencil, connect each box on the left with the appropriate box on the right.

| **Lead position** | **Lead** |
|---|---|

In the fourth intercostal space left sternal border

V1

In the fourth intercostal space right sternal border

V6

Anterior axillary line on the same horizontal plane as V4

V4

In the fifth intercostal space on the mid-clavicular line

V2

Midaxillary line on the same horizontal plane as V4

V5

**12** Label the following diagram:

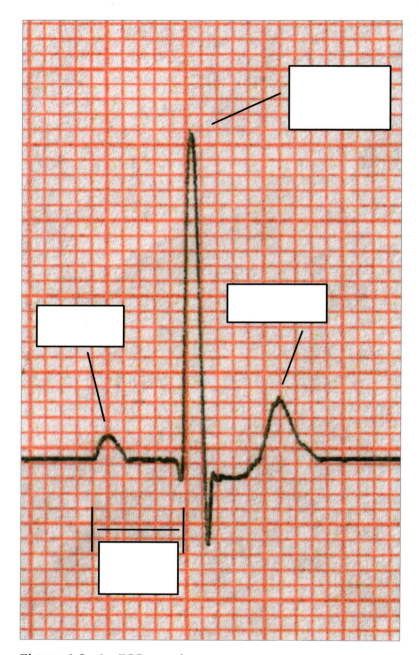

**Figure 4.8:** *An ECG complex*

# Chapter 5

# Common arrhythmias

A number of situations can arise that cause the normal heart rate to become too fast, too slow or irregular. These unusual patterns are referred to as arrhythmias. There are many different types of arrhythmia, with many different causes.

This chapter will explain five of the most common types of arrhythmia that you are likely to come across in practice: atrial fibrillation, atrial flutter, ventricular tachycardia, supraventricular tachycardia and ventricular fibrillation.

## Origin of arrhythmias

All arrhythmias originate somewhere in the heart's conduction system. The origin is called the focus (or foci, if there are several of them). It is fairly easy to see whether the focus of the arrhythmia is atrial or ventricular when you look at the ECG. As a rule, if the QRS complex is wide and abnormal to look at, the focus is in the ventricles. If the QRS is narrow, the focus is either in (or near) the AV node or in the atria.

## Atrial fibrillation

Atrial fibrillation (AF) is the most common cardiac arrhythmia. It is usually experienced by the elderly and those with heart failure, but it can occur at any age.

In AF the atria do not contract in their normal regular fashion, but instead 'twitch' rapidly and irregularly. These small, irregular contractions do not generate enough energy for the atria to pump blood into the ventricles, so blood pressure is often reduced as a result.

As we saw in Chapter 2, normal atrial conduction is shown on the ECG as a P wave that is small and rounded. This is because the SA node is solely responsible for the conduction of the atria. However, in AF many different parts of the atrial conduction system are conducting independently of each other, each trying to conduct the atria (see fig 5.1). On the ECG, it will look as if there is no P wave. Instead there will be a lot of chaotic activity on the baseline (see fig 5.2).

These fibrillations are so fast and irregular that the AV node is unable to pass all the conduction waves through into the ventricles. The AV node therefore only allows some of the conduction waves through. Because these atrial conductions are random, the conduction waves that do pass through the AV node are also irregular. This leads to an irregular heart rate.

On the ECG, the key features of AF are:

- absence of a P wave – showing that the atria are not being conducted from the SA node;
- chaotic activity on the baseline – from the multiple sources of conduction (or foci);
- irregular QRS rate – as the AV node tries to regulate the heart rate;
- narrow/unchanged QRS complexes – because the ventricular conduction system is not affected.

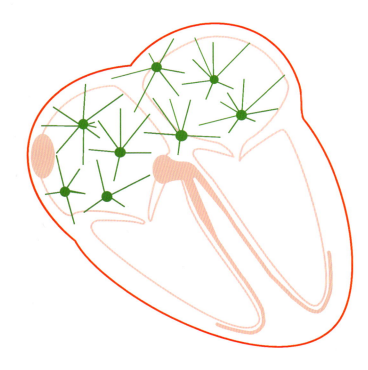

**Figure 5.1**
*Atrial fibrillation diagram.*

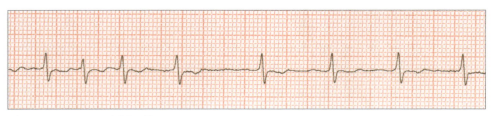

**Figure 5.2** *Atrial fibrillation ECG.*

AF can be fast or slow, or it might vary between fast and slow. The irregularity has no pattern (or cycle) to it, and each QRS complex will have a different interval between it and the next. This is sometimes referred to as 'irregularly irregular'.

## Atrial flutter

Like atrial fibrillation, atrial flutter is an arrhythmia in which the atria conduct very rapidly – more rapidly than the ventricles. The difference with atrial flutter is that there is only one focus in the atrium that is conducting quickly, rather than the multiple foci found in atrial fibrillation.

Because there is only one focus for this arrhythmia, it is possible to see some rough-looking waves on the baseline. These are called flutter waves and they tend to be tall, broad and 'sawtooth' shaped (see fig 5.3). You will notice that when one flutter wave ends, another starts straight away. This is because the circuit that develops in the atria continuously conducts the atria, without a pause (see fig 5.4).

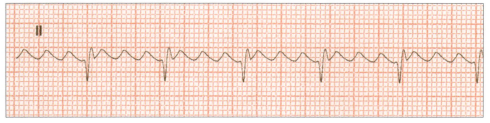

**Figure 5.3** *Atrial flutter ECG.*

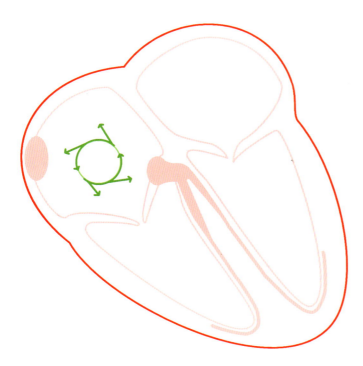

**Figure 5.4** *Atrial flutter diagram.*

The rate of these flutter waves is about 300 per minute. If all these conduction waves were transferred through to the ventricles, we would see a heart rate of 300, which would certainly lead to loss of consciousness. Thankfully, the AV node does its best to control the heart rate, and does not allow every flutter wave to pass through to the ventricles.

There is some variation in how often the AV node allows these conductions to pass into the ventricles. The ratio of flutter waves to each QRS complex may be 2:1, 3:1 or 4:1.

> **REMEMBER:**
>
> If this seems a little complicated, try thinking of these two arrhythmias as fireworks!
>
> Atrial fibrillation is like rockets going off at a firework party. At any one time, there may be many rockets exploding in the sky, sending out sparks in all directions. In the atria, many foci are going off like rockets, sending out waves of conduction in different, random and unpredictable directions.
>
> Atrial flutter is more like a catherine wheel, nailed to a post. It remains in one place but spins around very quickly, throwing out sparks in all directions each time it goes round. There is a more even pattern to the conduction in the atria because it is all coming from one place.

## Supraventricular tachycardia

Supraventricular tachycardia (SVT) is the name given to a whole range of arrhythmias, each with different causes. Their one common characteristic is that they all have their focus above the ventricles, as the name implies.

SVT may be a result of the SA node conducting too quickly, or because of some genetic conduction disorder. Most commonly, SVT comes about as a result of some interruption or disturbance to some of the conduction tissue near (or sometimes inside) the AV node. This is referred to as AV nodal re-entry tachycardia (AVNRT).

In this case, a small circuit develops in the conduction tissue that rapidly generates ventricular conductions (see fig 5.6). The circuit acts in a similar way to that which causes atrial flutter (see above).

Each time the conduction completes one circuit, a wave of conduction is sent off into the ventricles. However, unlike atrial flutter, the AV node is unable to regulate the heart rate, so each circuit results in a QRS complex.

The key ECG features of SVT are therefore:

● narrow QRS – because the conduction moves through the ventricles normally;

● P wave present but sometimes not visible if the heart rate is too high;

● regular but rapid heart rate.

SVT may come in short bursts or may be sustained for some time. The patient may have low blood pressure, shortness of breath and/or chest pain, or may lose consciousness.

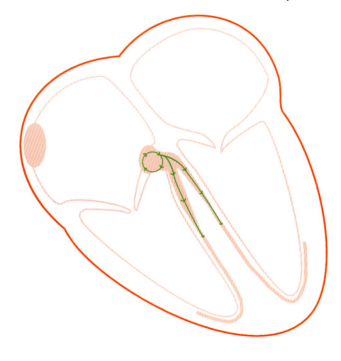

**Figure 5.5**:
*Supraventricular tachycardia diagram.*

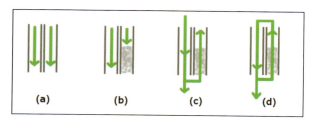

**Figure 5.6** *SVT conduction circuit.*

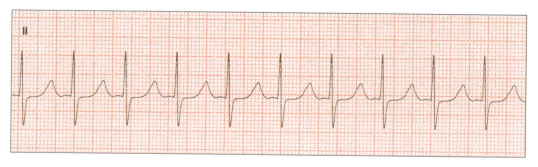

**Figure 5.7** *Supraventricular tachycardia ECG.*

## Ventricular tachycardia

Ventricular tachycardia arises from the ventricular conduction system. Its focus is usually an area of conduction tissue that has been affected by cellular injury or by some local electrolyte changes. The mechanism is often similar to the AVNRT (see p. 29). A small circuit develops in the conduction fibres and leads to a rapid cycle of conduction occurring across the ventricles (see fig 5.8).

Because the normal conduction system through the ventricles is not being used, the wave of conduction takes much longer to travel across the ventricular mass. This explains why the resulting QRS complex is broad and abnormally shaped (see fig 5.9).

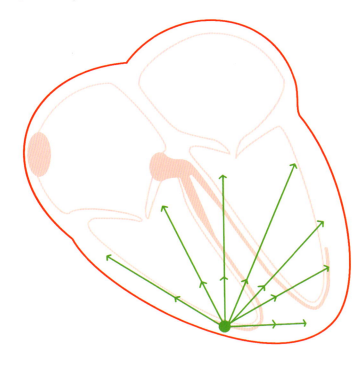

**Figure 5.8**
*Ventricular tachycardia diagram.*

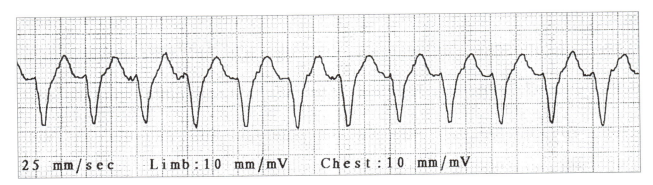

25 mm/sec     Limb:10 mm/mV     Chest:10 mm/mV

**Figure 5.9** *Ventricular tachycardia ECG.*

The key ECG features of ventricular tachycardia are:

● no P waves – or, if seen, they do not always immediately precede a QRS;

● broad QRS complexes;

● regular but rapid heart rate.

## Ventricular fibrillation

Ventricular fibrillation (VF) is a life-threatening arrhythmia and the patient requires immediate medical attention.

As with atrial fibrillation, there are multiple foci in the ventricles that are all discharging

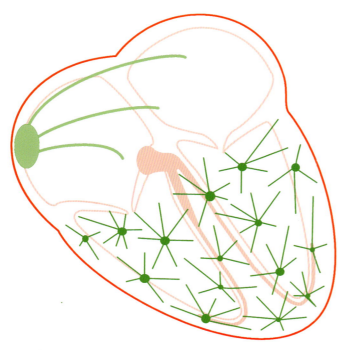

**Figure 5.10**

*Ventricular fibrillation – multiple foci within the Purkinje system simultaneously attempt to depolarise the ventricles.*

simultaneously (see fig 5.10). There is no coordinated electrical conduction within the ventricles; and the ventricular myo-cardium twitches chaotically, rather than contracting. The heart has essentially stopped.

If your patient is still conscious, then this is not VF, and you should check the equipment and electrodes.

VF can be Fine or Coarse but both types represent a cardiac arrest situation and should be treated accordingly.

The key ECG features of ventricular fibrillation are:

- no P waves;
- no QRS complexes;
- chaotic activity on the baseline;
- may be coarse or fine.

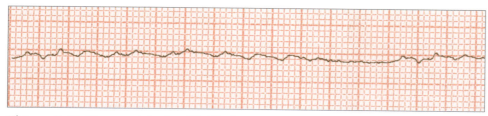

**Figure 5.11** *Fine ventricular fibrillation.*

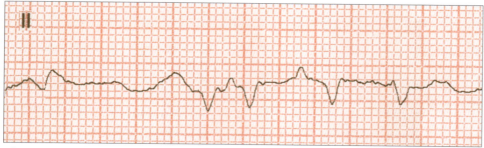

**Figure 5.12** *Coarse ventricular fibrillation.*

# Chapter 5 activities

The following exercise will test your recognition of the common arrhythmias covered in this chapter.

### Activity 5.1: Recognising different arrhythmias

*Approximate time required to complete this activity: 5 minutes.*

*Answers are provided on p. 91.*

On the left is a description of an ECG rhythm; on the right is a list of arrhythmias. Tick the box in the middle column next to the arrhythmia that you feel fits the description best.

| | **Description** | **Tick** | **Arrhythmia** |
|---|---|---|---|
| **A** | No P waves<br>Broad complex<br>Heart rate 160 | | Atrial fibrillation |
| | | | Atrial flutter |
| | | | Supraventricular tachycardia |
| | | | Ventricular tachycardia |
| | | | Ventricular fibrillation |
| **B** | Heart rate 150<br>Broad, abnormal waves on the baseline<br>Normal QRS complexes | | Atrial fibrillation |
| | | | Atrial flutter |
| | | | Supraventricular tachycardia |
| | | | Ventricular tachycardia |
| | | | Ventricular fibrillation |
| **C** | Chaotic electrical activity on the baseline<br>No QRS complexes<br>No P waves seen | | Atrial fibrillation |
| | | | Atrial flutter |
| | | | Supraventricular tachycardia |
| | | | Ventricular tachycardia |
| | | | Ventricular fibrillation |
| **D** | Irregular heart rate<br>No P waves seen<br>Narrow QRS complexes | | Atrial fibrillation |
| | | | Atrial flutter |
| | | | Supraventricular tachycardia |
| | | | Ventricular tachycardia |
| | | | Ventricular fibrillation |
| **E** | Heart rate 180<br>Narrow QRS complexes<br>P wave not seen (might be hidden in the T wave of the preceding complex) | | Atrial fibrillation |
| | | | Atrial flutter |
| | | | Supraventricular tachycardia |
| | | | Ventricular tachycardia |
| | | | Ventricular fibrillation |

# Chapter 6

# Ectopics and extrasystoles

Ectopic beats are extra heartbeats that arise from a focus other than the sino-atrial node and occur early in the cardiac cycle. They are also commonly referred to as extrasystoles or premature contractions.

## Ventricular ectopics

Ventricular ectopics are early beats that begin in the ventricles and appear as wide, bizarre complexes (see fig 6.1). They tend to be followed by a compensatory pause, and are not always preceded by a P wave.

The wide, bizarre-looking shape is due to the early impulse beginning in one ventricle and spreading to the other but with some delay. This delay occurs because the impulse is conducted more slowly through the ventricles than through normal conduction pathways.

Meanwhile, the atrial cycle continues independently. No ectopic P wave is present. A P wave may occur either directly before or after the QRS but does not bear any relationship to it.

The pause following the ectopic is called 'a compensatory pause' because the cycle following the ectopic is compensating for the prematurity of the beat. The sinus rhythm resumes again as scheduled.

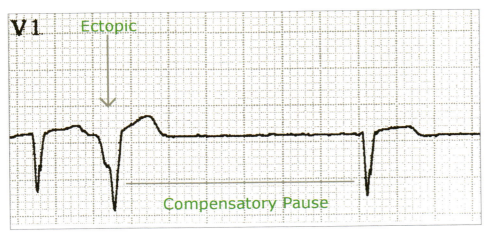

**Figure 6.1**
*A ventricular ectopic (originating from the left ventricle), followed by a compensatory pause.*

Ventricular ectopics may be isolated or may be a few in a row. More than six ventricular ectopics in a row constitute a ventricular tachycardia (see Chapter 5).

Ventricular ectopics may be positive or negative complexes. To find out which they are, you need to view lead V1 of your ECG or rhythm strip. If in V1 the QRS complex of the ectopic is positive, the impulse must be travelling towards the right and therefore coming from the left. If the QRS complex of the ectopic is negative, the impulse must be travelling towards the left and therefore coming from the right.

When some ectopics seen on a rhythm strip are positive and some are negative, they are collectively referred to as multifocal ectopics.

Bigeminy is a term used to describe an arrhythmia in which every other beat is a ventricular ectopic.

Isolated ventricular ectopics have little effect on the pumping action of the heart and usually do not cause symptoms, unless they are frequent. The main symptom is the feeling of the heart 'skipping a beat'. They tend not to be dangerous for people who do not have a heart disorder. However, when they occur frequently in people who have structural heart disease, they may be followed by life-threatening arrhythmias such as ventricular tachycardia and ventricular fibrillation (see Chapter 5).

When a ventricular ectopic falls so early that it interrupts the T wave of the preceding complex there is a high risk of ventricular tachycardia or fibrillation. The apex of the T wave is a vulnerable phase in the ventricular cycle. If stimulated by an ectopic, it may produce repeated ventricular responses, leading to these life-threatening arrhythmias. This is known as the R on T phenomenon.

The most common causes of ventricular ectopics are hypokalaemia and ischaemia, particularly in the early stages of myocardial infarction, when the ventricles are irritable. Indeed if you watch a monitor of a patient who is starting to get ischaemic chest pain, it is common to see ventricular ectopics appearing on the tracing. Hypokalaemia can easily be corrected with oral or intravenous potassium supplements, aiming to keep the patient's level at around 4mmol/l.

Ventricular ectopics are not usually treated if the patient is asymptomatic, as anti-arrhythmic drugs can also be pro-arrhythmic. These medications should therefore only be used for patients with symptoms.

## Atrial ectopics

Atrial ectopics are premature contractions that originate in the atria but not in the SA node. The atria are depolarised from a different direction from normal. The ectopic P wave therefore has a different shape (or morphology) from the sinus P wave.

Sometimes the ectopic P wave gets caught in the T wave of the preceding beat, and this causes it to distort the shape of the T wave. At other times, if the ectopic originates near the AV node, the P wave is inverted or even absent. Ventricular depolarisation continues as usual, inscribing a normal width QRS complex.

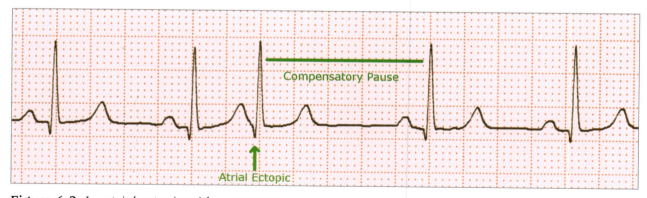

**Figure 6.2** *An atrial ectopic with a compensatory pause.*

Atrial ectopics may appear in isolation or there may be a few in a row, which then go on to develop into an atrial arrhythmia.

Infrequent or isolated atrial ectopics do occur in healthy individuals and are usually clinically insignificant. However, if the ectopics are becoming frequent this may indicate the onset of an atrial arrhythmia. Other causes of atrial arrhythmia can include: anxiety; stimulants such as caffeine, alcohol and excessive smoking; atrial hypertrophy; thyrotoxicosis and electrolyte disturbances.

Atrial ectopics do not usually require treatment.

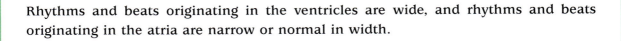

> **REMEMBER:**
>
> **Rhythms and beats originating in the ventricles are wide, and rhythms and beats originating in the atria are narrow or normal in width.**

# Chapter 6 activities

### Activity 6.1: Identifying origins of ectopics

*Approximate time required to complete this activity: 10 minutes*

*Answers are provided on p. 91.*

Look at the three rhythm strips below. Identify any ectopic beats and state where in the heart they originate.

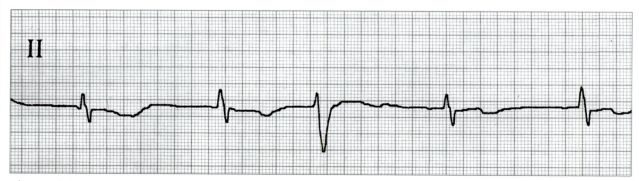

**Figure 6.3a**

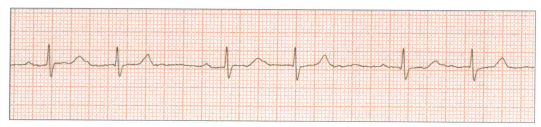

**Figure 6.3b**

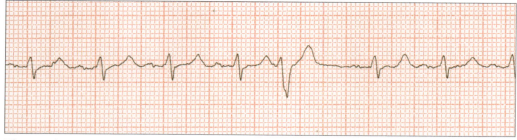

**Figure 6.3c**

Chapter 7

# The 12 lead ECG

So far we have discussed examining heart rhythms on single rhythm strips. The 12 lead ECG (see fig 7.1 below) provides additional diagnostic information because it records the electrical activity of the heart from three directions, whereas a single rhythm strip examines the heart from only one direction. With a 12 lead ECG, electrodes are placed on various sites of the body and each site gives a different view of the heart's electrical impulses. Each view of the heart is known as a lead.

If we look at Figure 7.1, the leads on the left-hand side of the page above the rhythm strip (i.e. those labelled I, II, III, aVR, aVL and aVF) are collectively known as the *limb leads*. Those on the right-hand side of the page (labelled V1–V6) are collectively known as the *chest leads*.

When we looked at rhythm strips earlier, we saw what a rhythm strip should look like in normal circumstances. This made it easier to go on and identify abnormalities on rhythm strips. We will take the same approach now with the 12 lead ECG, starting with normal readings and going on to look at abnormal readings.

## The limb leads (I, II, III, aVR, aVL and aVF)

If we look at the limb leads we see that some of the QRS complexes are positive (pointing upwards) and some are negative (pointing downwards). This is referred to as the polarity of the limb leads. We will now learn which ones should be positive and which ones should be negative.

> **REMEMBER:**
> **If an impulse travels towards an electrode, a positive QRS complex will be recorded.**
> **If an impulse travels away from an electrode, a negative QRS will be recorded.**

Figure 7.2 shows the position of the limb leads around the heart in relation to the pathway of the electrical impulse (as previously discussed on p. 4). We can see that the impulse is travelling directly towards Lead II and this is therefore the most positive QRS complex. This is why Lead II is often the lead that is produced on the ECG rhythm strip. It reflects the normal pathway of the impulse so it is usually the best lead to pick up the wave forms of the PQRST complex.

The impulse is travelling directly away from aVR and so this lead has a negative QRS complex. All the limb leads except aVR are positive, as the impulse is travelling in their direction. Some are more positive than others because the impulse travels more directly towards some electrodes than others.

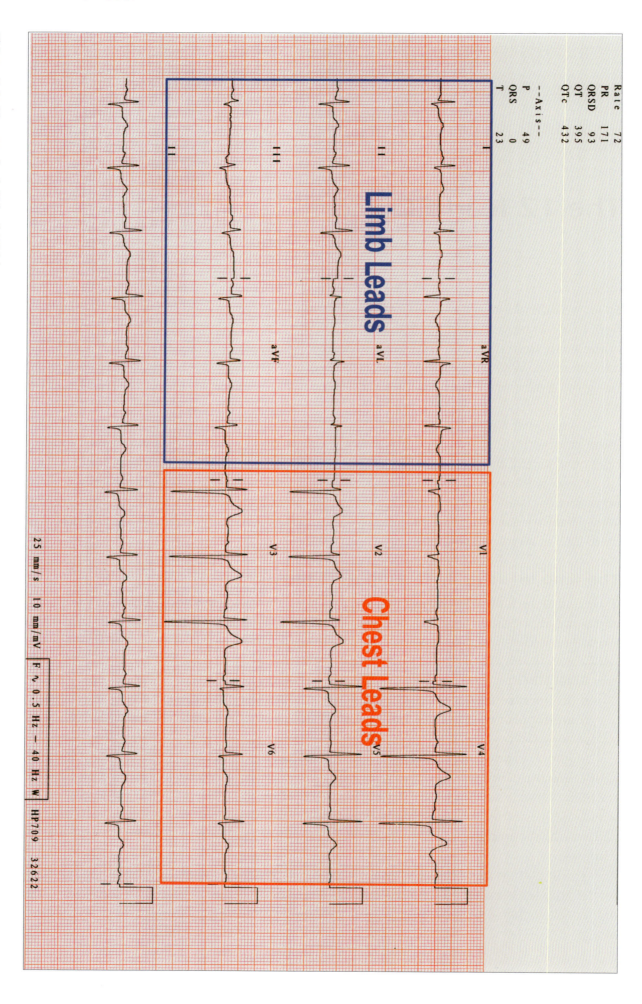

**Figure 7.1:** The standard 12 lead ECG layout.

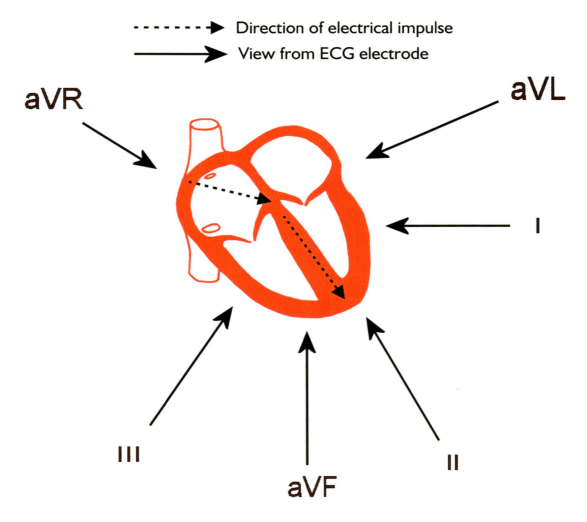

**- - - - - - ▶** Direction of electrical impulse

**───────▶** View from ECG electrode

**Figure 7.2:** *Views of the heart from the six limb leads.*

## SUMMARY:

In a normal ECG all the limb leads are positive, except aVR.

## The chest leads (V1–V6)

To understand what the chest leads should look like in a normal ECG, we need to start by looking back at the explanation of the QRS complex (see p. 8). QRS is in fact just a general term used for the ventricular part of the ECG complex. The way it is labelled actually depends upon the direction of the deflections.

The *first positive deflection* from the baseline is called an **R wave**.

The *first negative deflection* from the baseline is called a **Q wave**.

A *negative deflection* after an R wave is called an **S wave**.

It is possible to have more than one positive or negative deflection in a QRS complex. These are called R1 or S1 waves respectively.

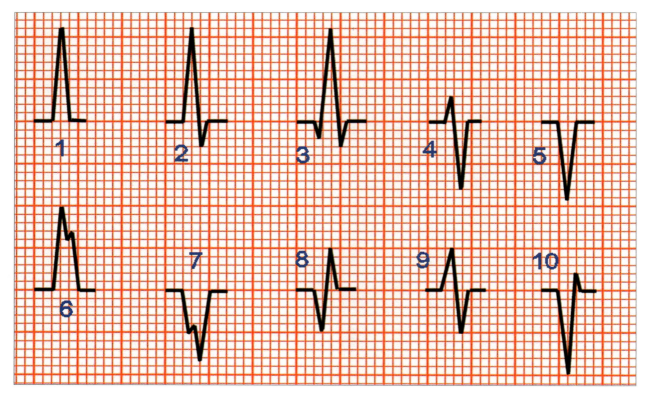

**Figure 7.3:** *Variations of the QRS complex: 1) R wave; 2) Rs complex; 3) qRs; 4) rS; 5) qS; 6) Rsr1; 7) QrS; 8) QR; 9) RS (Note that 8 and 9 are* **equiphasic***; they are as positive as they are negative); 10) Qr (Note that upper and lower case letters denote the relative size of the wave compared to the others in the complex).*

This knowledge helps us to identify how the chest leads look in a normal ECG. We look for **R wave progression.**

In V1 there should be a tiny R wave (positive deflection after the PR interval), in V2 this should be slightly bigger (i.e. progressing), in V3 bigger still, and then in V4 this should be the tallest R wave. In V5 and V6 the R waves should start to lose their height (see fig 7.4).

The ECG either shows good R wave progression (see fig 7.4) or poor R wave progression, where this pattern is not evident. If a lead has no R wave it has Q waves instead. As we will learn later (on p. 45), Q waves can indicate that the patient has had a heart attack in the past (see fig 7.5).

This pattern in the V leads can be explained by the way the directions of the electrical impulses depolarise the heart. As we saw earlier, if an impulse travels towards an electrode there is a positive deflection on the ECG and if the impulse travels away from the electrode there is a negative deflection.

When the impulse reaches the septum it **depolarises the septum from left to right**. This is because the impulse descends the left bundle branch more rapidly than the right. Both ventricles are activated simultaneously. However the wall of the right ventricle is much thinner than the left so the impulse travels through the right ventricular wall to the epicardium before the impulse on the left reaches the epicardium.

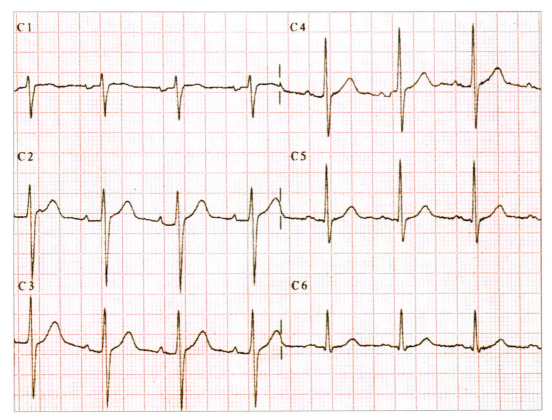

**Figure 7.4:** *Good R wave progression. The R wave becomes progressively taller from V1 to V4. The S wave becomes smaller until it disappears completely in V6. NB. Some ECG recorders label the chest leads C1–C6, rather than V1–V6, but they mean the same thing.*

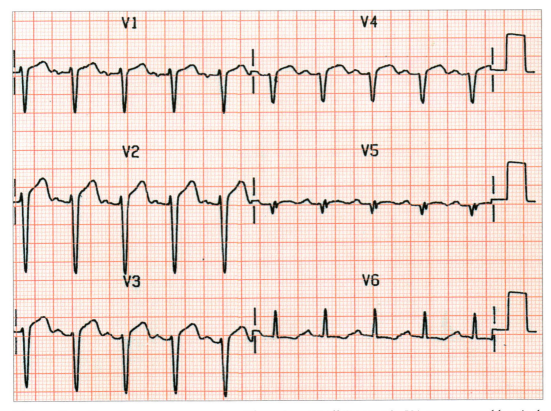

**Figure 7.5:** *Poor R wave progression. There is a small R wave in V1 as expected but it does not increase in size through successive leads. However, it does look normal in lead V6. The S wave is deep in leads V1 to V4 and only reduces in size by a small amount.*

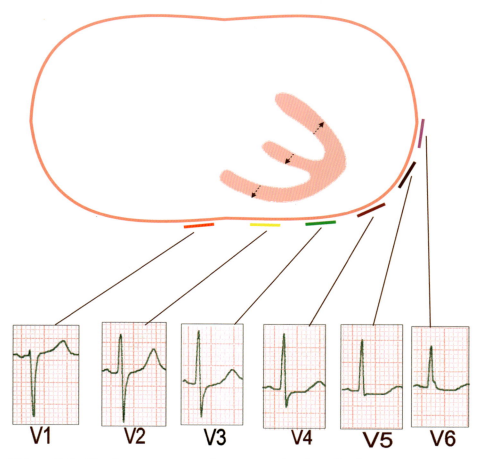

**Figure 7.6:** *The R wave progression across the chest leads.*

Figure 7.6 shows that if we are looking at V1 when the septum depolarises from left to right, the impulse firstly travels towards the V1 electrode, producing an R wave. When the impulse reaches the right ventricle it is also travelling towards the V1 electrode and therefore increases the positive deflection. The next impulse activating the left ventricle is travelling away from V1 and therefore produces a negative deflection (an S wave). This explains why we get a small R wave in V1, followed by an S wave.

   The V2 electrode is closer to the septum. Therefore, as the initial impulse has less distance to travel to the electrode, the R wave is more positive. In V3 the electrode is closer still; and in V4, which is situated on the septum, you will find the tallest R wave. V5 and V6 sit on the left of the septum so the initial impulse is travelling away from the electrode. This results in a small negative deflection (Q wave) as the initial deflection.

> **REMEMBER:**
> **Look at the V leads for R wave progression.**

# Chapter 7 activities

Chapter 7 has introduced the concept of R wave progression and the way in which the QRS complex looks different according to which lead (or view of the heart) you are using. The following activities will reinforce this learning so that you are better able to recognise normal and abnormal QRS complexes.

When you have completed these two activities you should be able to:

● identify the normal QRS complexes of the chest leads and the limb leads;

● recognise a good R wave progression across the chest leads.

### Activity 7.1: R wave progression.

*Approximate time required to complete this activity: 5 minutes*
*Answers are provided on p.92.*

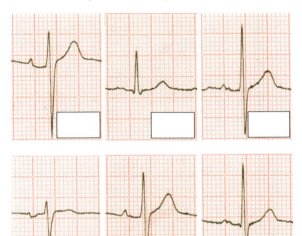

Look at these ECG complexes:

These are the six QRS complexes from the chest leads (V1–V6) on a normal ECG. They are presented here in the wrong order.

Using your knowledge of the normal R wave progression, label each complex with the appropriate label (V1, V2, V3, V4, V5 or V6).

### Activity 7.2: Identifying the components of the QRS complex on a 12 lead ECG

*Approximate time required to complete this activity: 10 minutes*

Get an ECG to look at.
(This could be the one that you took in Chapter 1 or any ECG that you have recorded since.)

Look at the QRS complex in each of the 12 leads and complete the following table:

| | I | II | III | aVL | aVR | aVF | V1 | V2 | V3 | V4 | V5 | V6 |
|---|---|---|---|---|---|---|---|---|---|---|---|---|
| Is this complex positive, negative or equiphasic? | | | | | | | | | | | | |
| Describe the complex (e.g. RS, QRS, etc) | | | | | | | | | | | | |
| Does this complex look as you would expect it to look? | | | | | | | | | | | | |

## Chapter 8

# Axis deviation

We have already learned about the normal pathway of the impulse as it travels through the conducting system. We have also seen how the direction of this impulse and the position of electrodes around the heart affect the polarity of the limb leads.

However, there may be times when the normal pathway of the impulse is disrupted, e.g. by a piece of damaged tissue as the result of a heart attack. Such a disruption may cause the pathway of the impulse to deviate to the left or the right or in extreme cases back up to the direction from which it came. This is known as *axis deviation*.

This disruption will affect the polarity of the limb leads. If something is causing the impulse to travel back from where it came, the aVR may be positive on the ECG, rather than negative, because the impulse is now travelling towards the aVR. Meanwhile Lead II may be negative, as the impulse is now travelling away from the lead.

One way of working out axis deviation is therefore by looking at the polarity of two of the limb leads. This can be most easily done by assessing Lead I and the aVF.

In a normal ECG, as we know, all the limb leads should be positive except aVR. Therefore, if the ECG shows a *normal axis deviation* (meaning that there is no disruption of the normal pathway of electrical activity) both *Lead I and the aVF should look positive* (see fig 8.1).

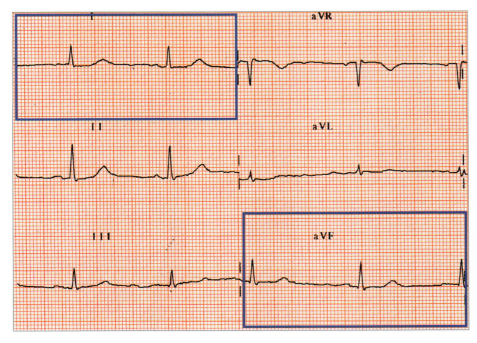

**Figure 8.1:** *Normal cardiac axis demonstrated by both Lead I and the aVF being positive.*

If there is an **extreme axis deviation** (severe disruption of the electrical pathway) the opposite will occur – *Lead I and the aVF will look negative* (see fig 8.2).

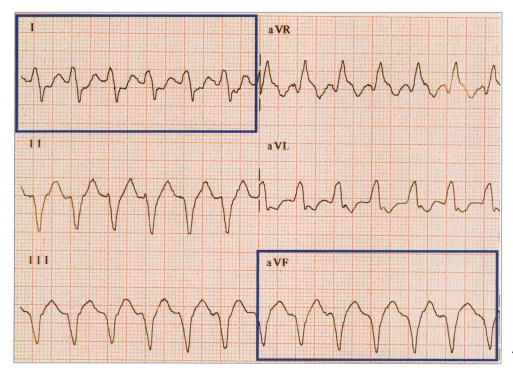

**Figure 8.2:**
*Extreme axis deviation. Lead I and the aVF lead are negative. Note that the aVR is positive; the electrical impulses are therefore moving in the opposite direction from normal.*

If the impulse deviates to the left, there is *left axis deviation, Lead I is positive and the aVF is negative*. This can be easily remembered by thinking about the tips of the QRS complexes of these two leads as leaving each other or leaving the page: *LEFT and LEAVING (start with the same letter!)* (see fig 8.3).

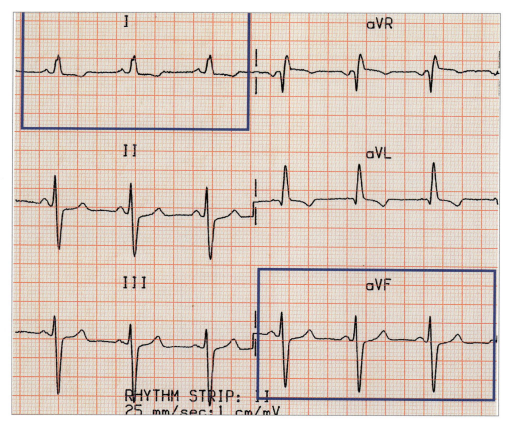

**Figure 8.3:**
*Left axis deviation. Lead I is positive and the aVF is negative.*

In *right axis deviation, Lead I is negative and the aVF is positive*. The tips of the QRS complexes reach for each other: *RIGHT and REACHING* (see fig 8.4).

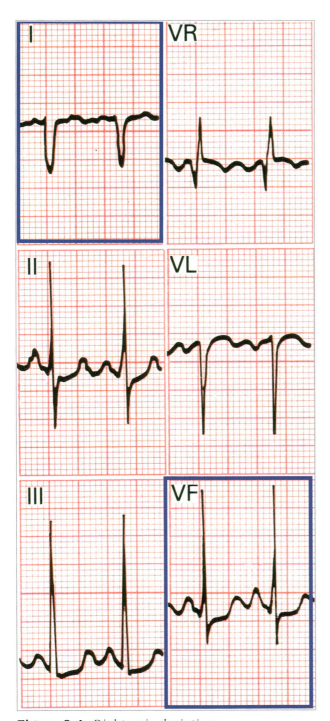

**Figure 8.4:** *Right axis deviation.*

Extreme axis deviation is the most worrying for a patient, then right axis deviation, and then left.

In practice, axis deviation does not necessarily require any treatment in itself. However, it raises the question of what has caused the axis deviation in the first place. For the clinician, the axis deviation will indicate how the patient's condition may be affecting the pathway of the impulse through the conducting system, and thus how likely the patient is to become unstable and have arrhythmias. Using the above method, axis deviation can be assessed at a glance as the ECG is coming out of the ECG machine.

## SUMMARY: Axis deviation

|          | I        | aVF            |
|----------|----------|----------------|
| Normal   | + ve     | + ve           |
| Left     | + ve     | -ve (leaving)  |
| Right    | -ve      | + ve (reaching)|
| Extreme  | -ve      | -ve            |

Occasionally, in more advanced cardiology, it may be necessary to talk about axis deviation in terms of degrees of deviation, rather than just in terms of normal, left, right or extreme. This can be done by plotting the axis on a graph called the Hexaxial Reference System (see fig 8.5). If an ECG shows a right axis deviation of +95 degrees, for example, it is not as serious as a right axis deviation of +170 degrees. The first method that we learned will be adequate for the majority of ECGs that you will encounter. However, calculating axis deviation using the Hexaxial Reference System is useful if you encounter a Lead I and aVF that are equiphasic (equally positive and negative). In addition, some complex arrhythmias can be distinguished from one another by the degree of axis deviation that is present.

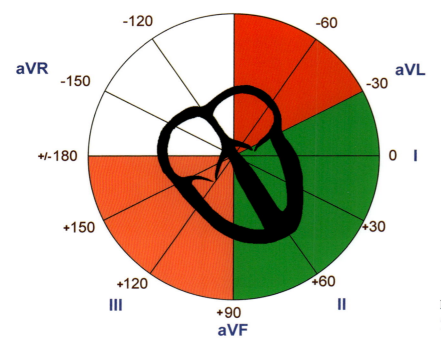

Figure 8.5:
*The Hexaxial Reference System.*

The purpose of including the Hexaxial Reference System within this text is simply to help make sense of what looks like a complex diagram in many ECG books. Such diagrams can make learners think they have reached their limit with ECG interpretation!

The Hexaxial Reference System is divided into 30-degree segments. The numbers at the bottom of the Hexaxial Reference System are positive and those at the top half, negative.

If you look at Figure 8.5 you will see which portion of the diagram represents which type of axis deviation. Here the heart is superimposed onto the Hexaxial Reference System. In normal circumstances, the pathway of the impulse would flow through the conducting system directly towards Lead II. This falls within the normal axis deviation quadrant of the Hexaxial Reference System. Anything deviating between +90 degrees and -30 degrees is considered normal axis deviation. If the pathway of the impulse deviates to the patient's left it would fall in the upper right-hand quadrant (as you look at the page) of the Hexaxial Reference System. If deviation is to the right, it would fall in the lower left-hand quadrant. And if the pathway of the impulse goes back to where it came from, it would travel towards the upper left quadrant, which represents extreme axis deviation.

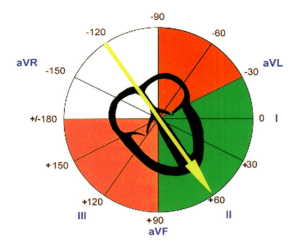

**Figure 8.5a:** *Normal electrical conduction; the impulses move towards Lead II.*

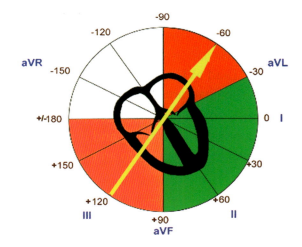

**Figure 8.5b:** *Left axis deviation; the impulses move in the approximate direction of Lead aVL.*

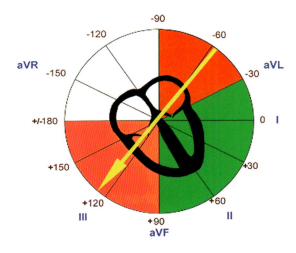

**Figure 8.5c:** *Right axis deviation; the impulses now move in the direction of Lead III.*

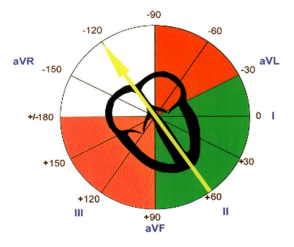

**Figure 8.5d:** *Extreme axis deviation; all electrical activity is moving in the opposite direction to normal.*

## Calculating axis deviation in degrees using the Hexaxial Reference System

Here is a step-by-step method to follow:

1 Look at the ECG and decide, by looking at Lead I and Lead aVF, if it is a normal, left, right or extreme axis deviation. If lead 1 is equiphasic (a complex that is as positive as it is negative), it is sufficient at this stage to say that it is either a left or a normal axis, for example.

2 Now look at the Hexaxial Reference System and remind yourself in which quadrant of the Reference System the axis will fall. (For instance, if it is a normal axis deviation it will fall between + 90 degrees and -30 degrees.)

3 Look back at the ECG and find the smallest, equiphasic complex (the smallest complex that is both positive and negative) in the limb leads. Remember: the smallest limb lead complex may not be equiphasic; you need to choose the lead that is both small and equiphasic.

**Activities 8**

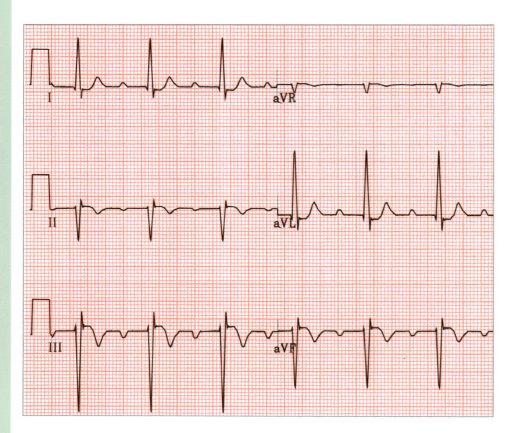

**Figure 8.8:** *ECG 2.*

Lead I is [       ] (positive or negative).

Lead aVF [       ] (positive or negative).

Therefore the axis is [     ] (left, right or normal).

Lead _____ is the smallest equiphasic lead. Lead _____ is 90 degrees to the most equiphasic lead.

Therefore, the cardiac axis is _____ degrees.

# Chapter 9

# Ischaemia, injury and necrosis

Animal experiments have played a major part in the development of ECG knowledge over the years. Fye (1994) describes how, as far back as 1790, Luigi Galvani used electrical stimulation to make a dead frog's leg dance. This was the first step in making a connection between electrical stimulation and the heart's contraction and it led on to the discovery of links between the heart's conducting system and myocardial contraction.

## Ischaemia

Much later, Bayley (1944) identified ECG changes by means of experiments performed on dogs. If a tourniquet is tied around a dog's coronary artery while it is connected to an ECG, and the coronary artery is **occluded** for a few minutes, a startling change occurs on the ECG trace. The T waves turn upside down (***T wave inversion***). This is known as an ***ischaemic change***. The term **ischaemia** refers to a condition where there is insufficient oxygenated blood reaching the myocardium (heart muscle). When the tourniquet is released the T waves turn upright again. Ischaemia is therefore a reversible change.

We can relate this to patients with angina. Angina is a condition in which the supply of blood to the myocardium does not match its demand for oxygen. The process may be reversed by giving the patient a tablet of Glyceryl trinitrate (GTN). GTN reduces the amount of blood flowing into the heart (its preload) and therefore lowers the heart's workload, reducing the myocardial need for oxygen – a similar effect to that gained by releasing the tourniquet.

There are two other ischaemic changes that we may see on an ECG: ***ST depression*** (where the second part of the QRS complex and the T wave are depressed below the baseline); and ***T wave flattening***.

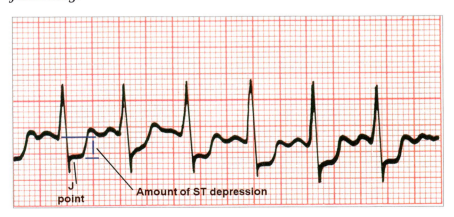

**Figure 9.1:** *ST depression. The amount of ST depression is measured from between the J point (the end of the S wave) and the* **isoelectric line**.

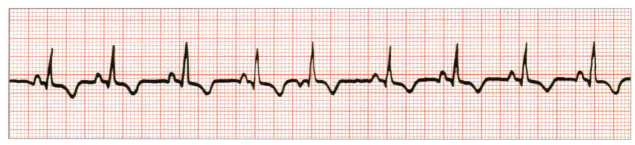

**Figure 9.2:** *T wave inversion.*

It is useful to record an ECG when a patient is experiencing chest pain. Often one of these ischaemic changes will be present and this may confirm that the patient's pain is cardiac in origin.

An exercise treadmill test is sometimes used to quantify a patient's symptoms during aerobic exercise. As the patient exerts themselves on the treadmill, the myocardium demands more oxygen and the patient may show symptoms. The development of ST depression on the ECG recorded during this procedure may indicate that the heart is becoming ischaemic, as the demand for oxygen increases with exercise. ST depression is measured from the bottom of the ECG's baseline to the ST segment.

## Injury

Following the Bayley experiment, scientists examined what would happen if the tourniquet was left on the dog's coronary artery a little longer. When this was tried, another startling change occurred. The second half of the QRS complex became elevated above the baseline. Known as ***ST elevation***, this is the change that is often seen when the patient is having a heart attack (acute myocardial infarction).

This is known as the ***injury*** stage and it can still be reversed if it is treated early enough. The supply of oxygen to the myocardium has been occluded and the occlusion therefore needs to be removed in order to reinstate the blood supply – again, like releasing the tourniquet. This is done by mechanically opening the vessel in a procedure called **primary angioplasty** and then inserting a coronary stent. This procedure is carried out in a specialist Angiography Suite. It is performed by introducing a catheter up through the femoral artery to the heart. This enables a balloon to be inflated in order to open up the artery. Alternatively, a metal structure (a stent) can be used to keep the artery open. The criteria for primary angioplasty are that the patient's ECG should show:

- 2 mm or more ST elevation in at least two chest leads;
- **or** 1 mm or more ST elevation in two or more of the limb leads (Springings *et al.* 1995);
- **or** have a posterior myocardial infarction (see Chapter 10);
- **or** new left bundle branch block (see Chapter 11).

The longer the treatment is delayed, the more likely the myocardium is to die from lack of oxygen. This is why the public are being educated to report symptoms of chest pain and seek help early. Once they have called for help, the patient's transfer to hospital for primary angioplasty should be as quick as possible (the 'call-to-balloon' time). The time between their arrival at hospital and the time they receive their primary angioplasty should also be as quick as possible (the 'door-to-balloon' time).

In the National Service Framework Document for Coronary Heart Disease (Department of Health 2000), the government has set targets to shorten these times in order to reduce deaths from coronary heart disease in the UK. The current target for door-to-balloon time is less than 2 hours (DANAMI-2 trial 2003).

- call-to-needle time should be less than one hour;
- door-to-needle time less than 20 minutes;
- and door-to-balloon time (in the case of primary angioplasty) less than two hours (DANAMI-2 trial, 2003).

## Necrosis

To continue with the Bayley experiment, our experimenters then wondered what would happen if the tourniquet was left on the dog's coronary artery for even longer? What happened was that after about six hours of occluding the blood supply to the myocardium, the myocardium started to die.

This is the **necrosis** (death) stage and manifests itself on the ECG by the development of deep **Q waves** (see fig 9.3).

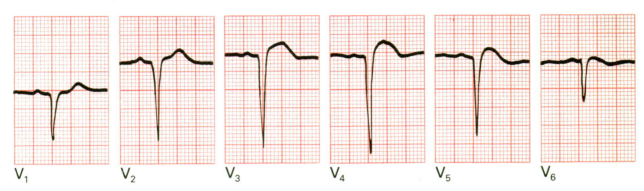

**Figure 9.3:** *Large Q waves on the ECG of a post-myocardial infarction patient.*

The necrosis stage is irreversible and this is what we want to avoid for our patients. Once myocardium is dead, it cannot be salvaged. The more necrosis occurs, the poorer the prognosis for the patient. This is why early **reperfusion** is vital. Once Q waves develop on an ECG, they stay there. Therefore, it is sometimes difficult, without an old ECG, or a sound patient history, to ascertain whether a patient's infarction is six hours old or considerably older!

We have already learned that it is normal to have Q waves in some leads. For Q waves to indicate necrosis (or be pathological), they have to be 25% of the height of the R wave or 2 mm in depth.

In time, T wave inversion then occurs in the leads with the Q waves and the ST elevation returns to baseline, leaving the T wave inverted. This is often referred to as the evolving pattern of myocardial infarction (see fig 9.4).

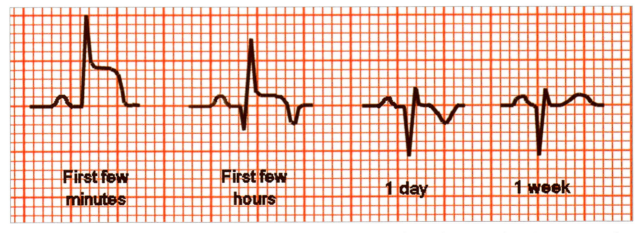

**Figure 9.4:** *The evolution of an acute myocardial infarction. In the early stages there is no Q wave but there is ST elevation. In the first few hours the Q wave develops and the T wave becomes inverted. If reperfusion of the affected artery does not take place then the myocardium becomes irreversibly damaged and this is shown as a large Q wave. At this stage the T wave is still inverted because the area around the necrosed myocardium is ischaemic. Over the coming weeks and months the necrosed tissue solidifies into scar tissue and the ischaemic zone around it develops new blood vessels; the Q wave remains a permanent feature of the ECG but the T wave will become positive again.*

## Non ST segment elevation myocardial infarction

Infarction may be limited to the inner part of the ventricular walls rather than the full thickness of the myocardium, or it can simply result in microscopic myocardial damage. In this case repolarisation is affected but not depolarisation; and the ECG will show deep, symmetrical **T wave inversion** or **ST depression**, rather than ST elevation and Q waves. Therefore, these types of infarcts are often referred to as **non ST elevation infarcts** (see fig 9.5). The difference between the T wave inversion in ischaemia and T wave inversion in the non Q wave myocardial infarction is that the T waves stay inverted rather than reverting to normal when the patient's symptoms improve.

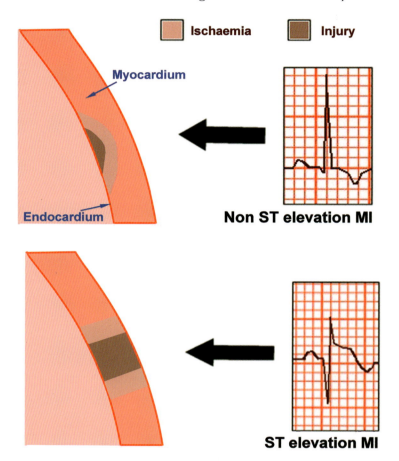

**Figure 9.5:** *The effects of ST and non ST elevation myocardial infarction (MI) on the ECG complex. The ST elevation MI is associated with myocardial injury that extends from the endocardium to the epicardium. The ECG shows ST elevation from the injured tissue and a large Q wave as a result of the developing necrosis. The non ST elevation MI only affects a portion of the endocardium and the ECG shows the ischaemic changes (T wave inversion) from the surrounding tissue.*

## Patient risk stratification

The term **acute coronary syndrome** is used to refer to several conditions within a spectrum of the same disease process. The extent to which these physical changes reduce the flow of blood through the coronary artery determines the exact nature of the clinical acute coronary syndrome that ensues. Acute coronary syndrome comprises:

● unstable angina;

● non ST segment elevation myocardial infarction (NSTEMI);

● Q wave myocardial infarction.

In the last few years much has changed in Cardiology in terms of how patients are risk stratified. An example of this is the use of **troponin** testing as a biochemical marker of myocardial damage. The presence of ST elevation in acute myocardial infarction is only about 50% sensitive (Rude *et al.*, 1983). Not all patients who develop myocardial necrosis exhibit ECG changes. Thus, a normal ECG does not rule out a diagnosis of myocardial infarction.

Troponins are contractile proteins that are present in heart muscle cells and leak into the patient's bloodstream during even minor myocardial injury (Adams *et al.*, 1993). In addition, they may predict cardiac events in patients with acute coronary syndromes. It is now clear that any amount of myocardial damage, as detected by cardiac troponins, implies an impaired clinical outcome for the patient, whatever the ECG reading (Antman *et al.*, 1996).

As stated by the Resuscitation Council UK: 'In the context of unstable angina, an elevated troponin level at 6–8 hours after pain indicates a higher risk of further coronary events than if the troponin level is normal (i.e. undetectable). A combination of ST depression on the ECG and a raised troponin identifies a particularly high risk group for subsequent myocardial infarction and sudden death.' (Resuscitation Council UK, 2005, p. 18)

Increasing acute chest pain admissions to hospital in the UK continue to stretch limited resources in Coronary Care units. There is therefore an urgent need to discriminate rapidly between high-risk and low-risk patients.

### Differential diagnosis

Differential diagnosis is made more difficult because many ECG changes sometimes, but ***do not always***, indicate acute coronary syndrome. Here are some examples:

- QS complexes occasionally occur in V1 and V2 as a normal variant in tall, thin individuals because of the positional changes of the electrodes relative to the heart.
- Persistent ST elevation in the chest leads often indicates formation of a ventricular **aneurysm**.
- Peaked T waves are characteristic of **hyperkalaemia** and flat T waves of **hypokalaemia**.
- T wave inversion is a normal variant in leads V1, V2, and V3 in Afro-Caribbean individuals.
- Concave ST elevation, with widespread T wave inversion occurs with **pericarditis**.
- Deep, inverted T waves are sometimes found after intracerebral bleeds.
- Similar T wave changes are often seen after **tachyarrhythmias** or Stokes–Adams attacks.

## SUMMARY:

- Ischaemia – T wave inversion, ST depression, T wave flattening
- Injury – ST elevation
- Necrosis – Q waves

*Caution:* It is possible for the ECG to be normal during a myocardial infarction or for other conditions to cause these changes. Therefore the ECG should **never** be used in isolation.

# Chapter 9 activities

When you have completed the following activity, you should be able to recognise the ECG changes associated with:

- myocardial ischaemia;
- myocardial injury;
- and myocardial necrosis.

### Activity 9.1: Recognising abnormalities associated with acute coronary syndrome

*Approximate time required to complete this activity: 15 minutes*
*Answers are provided on p. 93.*

Look at Figure 9.6 (opposite), which shows a 12 lead ECG with a number of abnormal changes on it. Then complete the following table:

| ECG lead | N for 'no' or Y for 'yes', as appropriate | | | | | |
|---|---|---|---|---|---|---|
| | Q waves? | ST elevation? | ST depression? | T wave inversion? | T wave flattening? | Likely cause/s (ischaemia, injury, necrosis) |
| I | | | | | | |
| II | | | | | | |
| III | | | | | | |
| aVR | | | | | | |
| aVL | | | | | | |
| aVF | | | | | | |
| V1 | | | | | | |
| V2 | | | | | | |
| V3 | | | | | | |
| V4 | | | | | | |
| V5 | | | | | | |
| V6 | | | | | | |

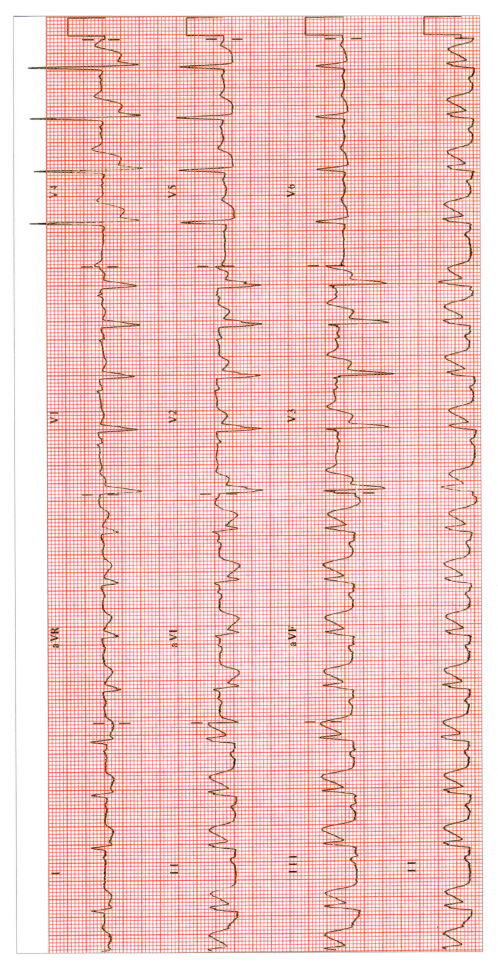

**Figure 9.6:** *A 12 lead ECG with a number of abnormal ECG changes on it.*

# Chapter 10

# Sites of infarction

Now that you know what changes you are looking for on the ECG, you need to learn which lead looks at which region of the heart. You can then put these two pieces of information together to help determine what is wrong with the patient and which part of the heart is affected.

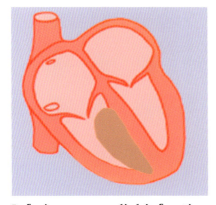

**Inferior myocardial infarction**

ST elevation in leads:

II

III

aVF

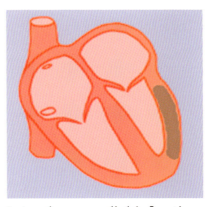

**Lateral myocardial infarction**

ST elevation in leads:

V5 & V6

I

aVL

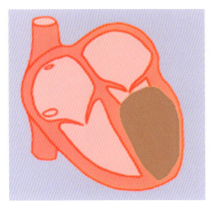

**Anterior myocardial infarction**

ST elevation in leads:

V1–6

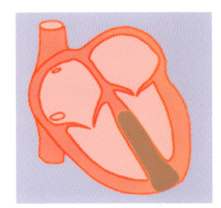

**Septal myocardial infarction**

ST elevation in leads:

V3–V4

**Figure 10.1:** *The leads of the 12 lead ECG and the surfaces of the heart. These are the four regions in which damage most commonly occurs during myocardial infarction. They can be recognised on the ECG by ST elevation in the leads that are closest to these regions.*

Looking at the left ventricle, we can label the different walls of this chamber: anterior, posterior, inferior and lateral.

- The **front** surface of the left ventricle is referred to as the **anterior** surface.
- The **bottom** part of the left ventricle is the **inferior** surface.
- The **back** of the left ventricle is the **posterior** surface.
- The **side** of the left ventricle is the **lateral** surface.

The changes described in Chapter 9 will appear in those ECG leads facing the area of ischaemia, injury or necrosis.

## Anterior leads

**V1 to V6** are generally known as the **anterior** leads. You can remember this by reminding yourself that the V leads are the ones you put across the front (or anterior aspect) of the chest when you take an ECG recording. ST elevation in these leads would be called an acute anterior myocardial infarction (see fig 10.2). To be more specific, **V1 and V2** look at the right ventricle; and **V3 and V4** look at the **septum**.

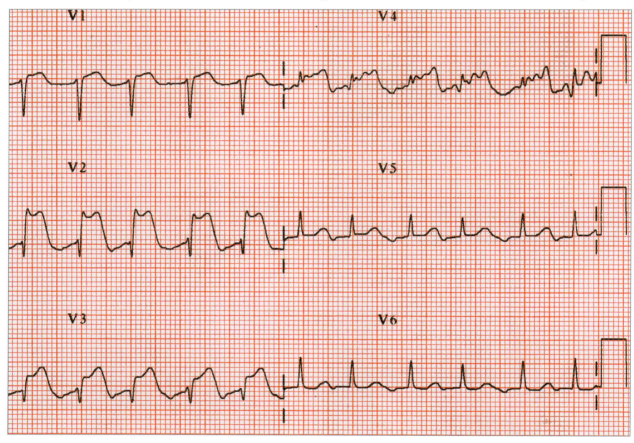

**Figure 10.2:** *Acute anterior myocardial infarction.*

## Inferior leads

**Leads II, III and aVF** are the **inferior leads**. ST elevation in these leads would therefore be called an acute **inferior** myocardial infarction (see fig 10.3).

## Lateral leads

The **lateral leads** are **V5 and V6, I and aVL** (the latter two are often referred to as **high lateral leads**). If ST elevation occurs in these leads it is called an acute **lateral** myocardial infarction.

Sometimes combinations of leads are affected. For instance, ST elevation in II, III, aVF, V5 and V6 would be called an acute **inferior-lateral** myocardial infarction.

Due to its position, looking at the heart, we do not use aVR when searching for signs of ischaemia, injury or necrosis.

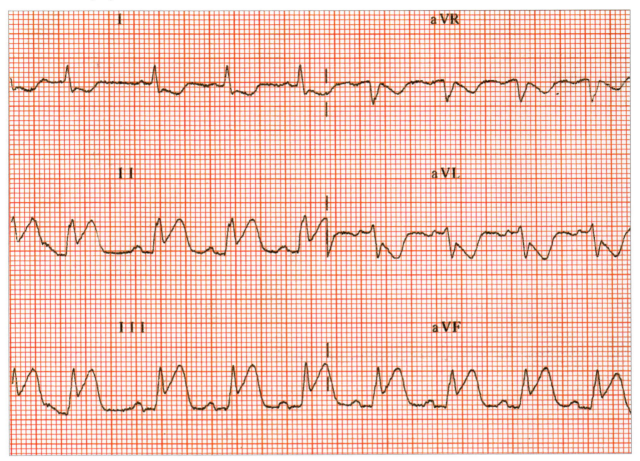

**Figure 10.3:** *Acute inferior myocardial infarction; ST elevation in Leads II, III and aVF.*

## Reciprocal changes

Figure 10.4, on page 66, shows that when there is ST elevation in one set of leads (i.e. the inferior leads), there is ST depression in the opposite set of leads (i.e. anterior) and the same the other way around. These changes are known as *reciprocal changes*.

## Coronary circulation

The site of the infarct can be determined by correlating the ECG findings with knowledge of the coronary circulation. However, normal coronary vasculature varies widely from individual to individual, so it is only possible to make generalisations. The two main coronary arteries are the right coronary artery and the left anterior descending coronary artery.

In most people, the right coronary artery supplies the right atrium, the right ventricle and the inferior part of the left ventricle. Therefore, occlusion of the right coronary artery can produce an inferior myocardial infarction. As blood supply to the right atrium is affected, ischaemia to the SA and AV nodes explains why **bradyarrhythmias** and heart blocks are often associated with inferior myocardial infarctions.

The left anterior descending coronary artery, in the majority of the population, supplies blood to the front of the left ventricular wall and the septum. If this artery is occluded, an anterior myocardial infarction usually results and is often complicated by impairment of the left ventricular function.

As you can see, having a knowledge of the ECG and the coronary circulation can often help you to predict the complications that might accompany the infarction and enable you to take preventative measures.

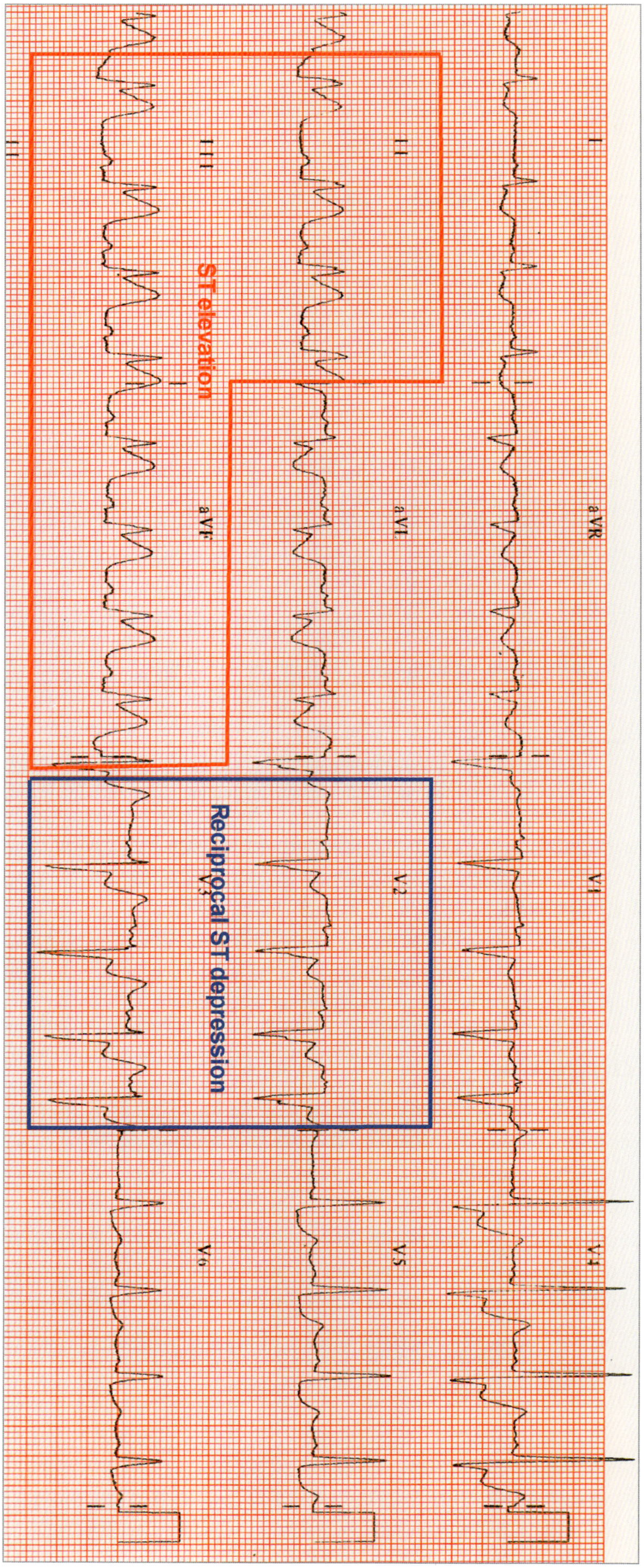

**Figure 10.4:** *Reciprocal changes: ST elevations in II, III and aVF indicate an acute inferior MI. Leads V2 and V3 are mirroring these changes in the inferior wall of the left ventricle.*

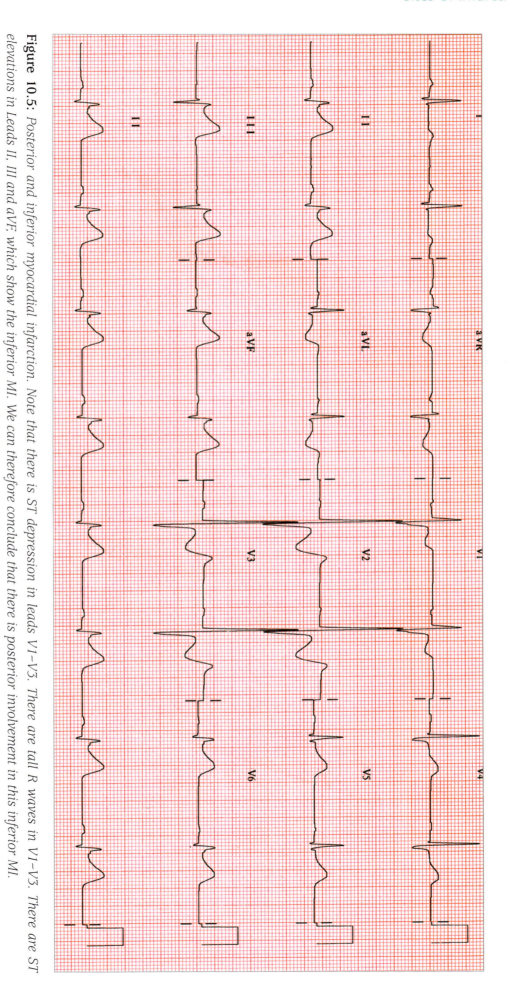

**Figure 10.5:** *Posterior and inferior myocardial infarction. Note that there is ST depression in leads V1–V3. There are tall R waves in V1–V3. There are ST elevations in Leads II, III and aVF, which show the inferior MI. We can therefore conclude that there is posterior involvement in this inferior MI.*

## Posterior myocardial infarction

We have not yet talked about posterior myocardial infarctions and we have used up all the leads from our 12 lead ECG! *Posterior* myocardial infarction is usually recognised when there is a reciprocal change in *V1 and V2* (see fig 10.5). For example, *ST depression* in these leads reflects posterior ST elevation and the development of an abnormally *tall R wave in V1 and V2* reflects posterior Q waves. The right coronary artery also supplies the blood to the posterior of the left ventricle. A posterior infarction can therefore be caused by an occlusion of the right coronary artery and is often accompanied by an inferior myocardial infarction. Posterior myocardial infarctions are slightly more difficult to recognise, and if they are overlooked the patient can miss out on the benefits of *revascularisation*.

## SUMMARY:

V1–V4            Anterior leads

II, III and aVF      Inferior leads

V5 , V6, I and aVL    Lateral leads

Always suspect a posterior infarct if the ECG shows tall R waves or ST depression in V1 and V2, especially if accompanied by an inferior myocardial infarction.

# Chapter 10 activities

It is very important to be familiar with the different surfaces of the heart when you are looking at ischaemia and infarction. The ECG changes associated with these conditions occur in very specific regions and these should be remembered. The activities for this chapter will reinforce your knowledge of how the ECG leads represent the different regions of the myocardium.

When you have completed these two activities, you should be able to:

- identify the ECG lead that shows each surface of the myocardium;
- recognise patterns of infarction and ischaemia on an ECG.

### Activity 10.1: The surfaces of the myocardium
*Approximate time needed to complete this activity: 5 minutes*
*Answers are provided on p. 93.*

Draw a line linking each box on the left with the appropriate box on the right.

**Myocardial region**                    **ECG leads**

| | |
|---|---|
| Anterior | ST elevation in II, III and aVF |
| Lateral | ST depression and tall R waves in V1–V2 |
| Inferior | ST elevation in V1–V6 |
| Septal | ST elevation in I, aVL V5–V6 |
| Posterior | ST elevation in V3–V4 |

Activities 10

**Activities 10**

### Activity 10.2: Recognising infarction on the 12 lead ECG

*Approximate time required to complete this activity: 10 minutes*
*Answers are provided on p. 94.*

Look at the two 12 lead ECGs shown in Figures 10.6 and 10.7 (pages 71 and 72). Can you identify the location of the infarction in both cases?

Make a note of any other abnormalities that you can see.

Activities 10

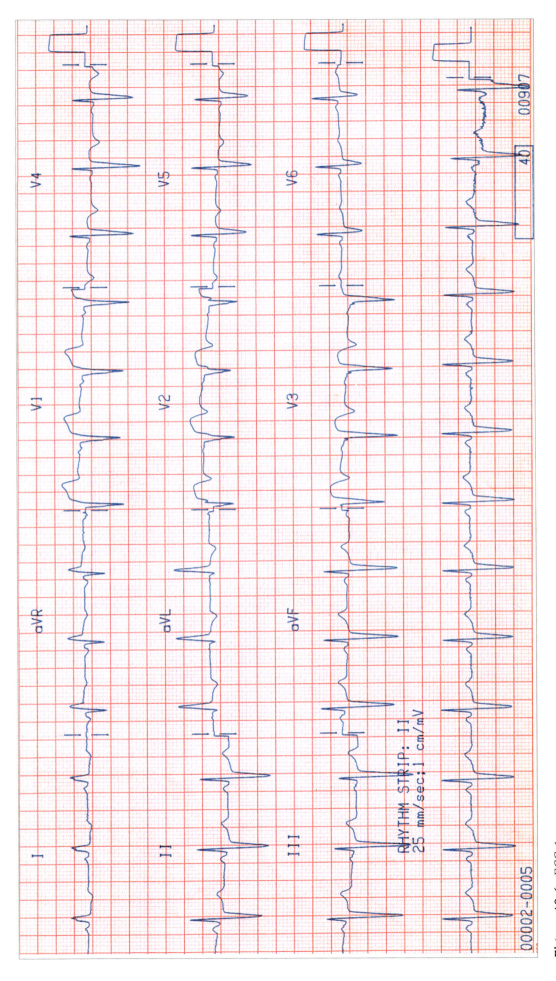

RHYTHM STRIP: II
25 mm/sec;1 cm/mV

00002-0005

**Figure 10.6:** *ECG 1.*

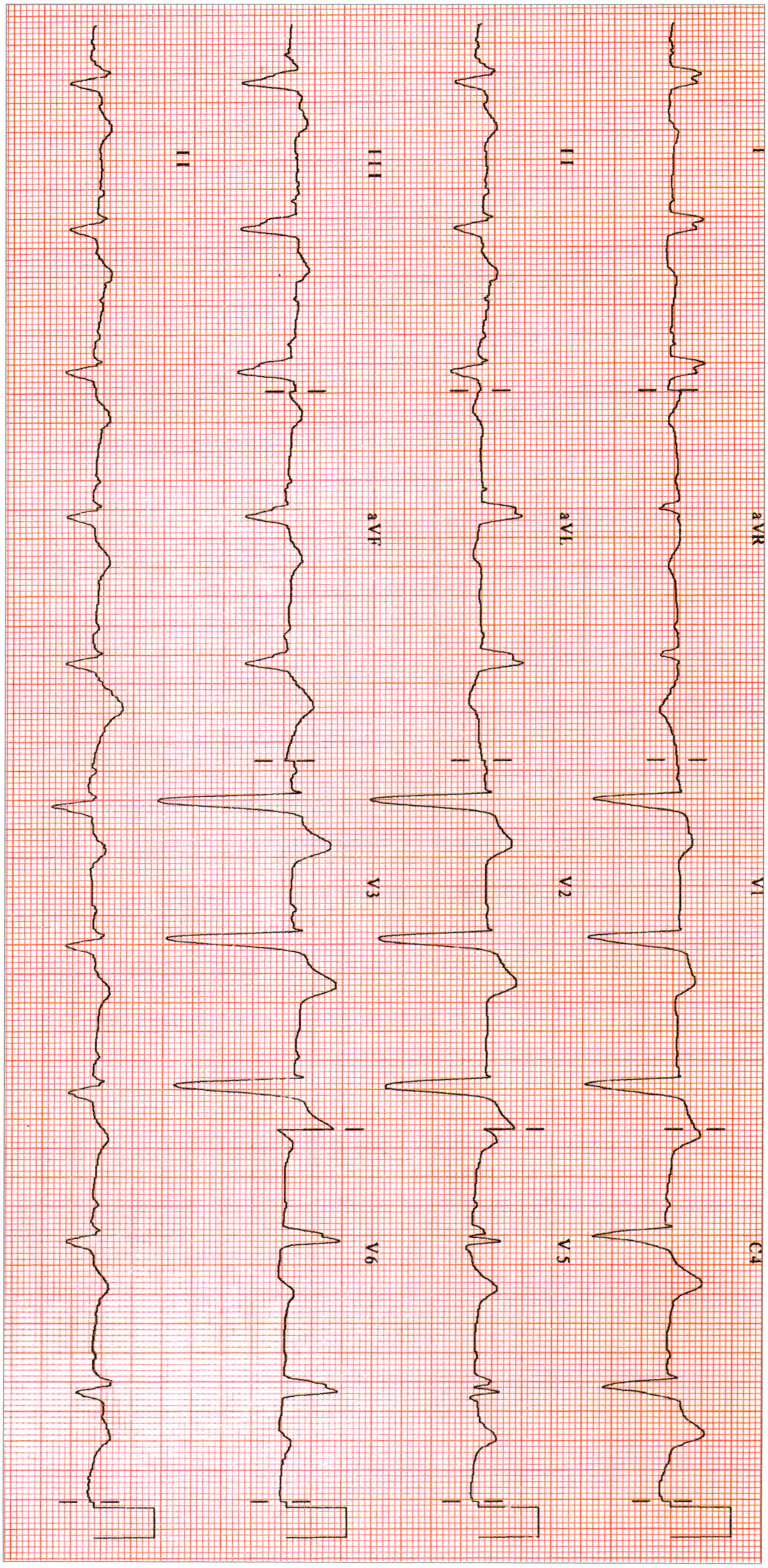

**Figure 11.2:** *Left bundle branch block ECG.*

As V6 sits opposite V1, it will be affected in the opposite way. Therefore the small Q waves that are usually seen in the lateral leads will not be evident. The entire QRS complex in left bundle branch block will be widened (greater than 0.12 seconds) owing to the conduction delay (see fig 11.2, page 62).

## Right bundle branch block

A delay or blockage of the conduction in the right bundle branch is called right bundle branch block. A normal impulse is initiated in the SA node and causes the atria to depolarise. The impulse then travels through the AV node and reaches the bundle branches. If the right bundle branch is blocked, the impulse will go down the left bundle branch. The initial activation in the ventricles remains the same as that in normal depolarisation (i.e. from left to right). Lead V1 will have an initial R wave inscribed, as the initial impulse is travelling towards that electrode. The left ventricle depolarises first and inscribes an S wave in V1, as the forces of depolarisation are now travelling away from V1. The right ventricle then depolarises. As the wave of depolarisation moves towards V1, an R' is inscribed. Again, the opposite pattern will be inscribed in V6 (see fig 11.3).

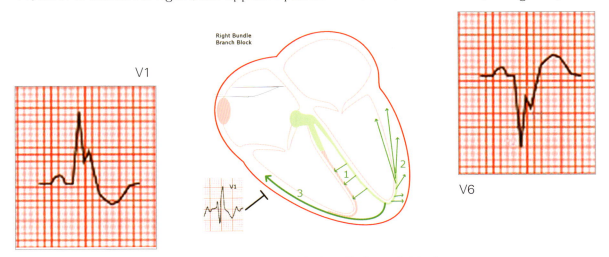

**Figure 11.3:** *The sequence of conduction in right bundle branch block.*

The entire QRS complex will be widened (greater than 0.12 seconds) owing to the conduction delay. Thus, the pattern of right bundle branch block is a broad positive complex in V1 (see fig 11.4, page 64).

A simple way of reminding yourself what left and right bundle branch block look like on an ECG is by remembering two words:

**WILLIAM**

**MARROW**

The letter 'L' in William represents left bundle branch block and the letter 'R' in Marrow represents right bundle branch block. The first letter of each word will tell you what V1 should look like on the ECG, i.e. in the left bundle branch block V1 should be broad and negative (like the W shape in William). Likewise, in the right bundle branch block V1 should be narrow and positive (like the M shape in Marrow).

## Clinical significance

In right bundle branch block the initial depolarisation pathway of the impulse is not altered, so the ECG signs of myocardial infarction are not obscured. However, this is not the case with left bundle branch block. This is another item that we could add to our list of factors that can mimic myocardial infarction on the ECG.

# Chapter 11 activities

In Chapter 11 you have seen that there are ECG patterns that indicate a conduction block in the bundle branches. These patterns can vary quite a lot and do not always look as you would expect. The following activity will give you an opportunity to examine some bundle branch block patterns that vary considerably from each other.

When you have completed this activity, you should be able to:

● recognise RSR and QRS patterns in a variety of ECG complexes;
● differentiate between right and left bundle branch block on a 12 lead ECG.

### Activity 11.1: Recognising RSR and QRS patterns

*Approximate time required to complete this activity: 5 minutes*
*Answers are provided on p. 94.*

Look at the ECG rhythm strips in Figure 11.5 and label the complexes on each: R, S, R1 or S1. In the boxes below the rhythm strips make notes about the complex (its width, whether it is positive or negative, etc.), then identify whether it is right or left bundle branch block.

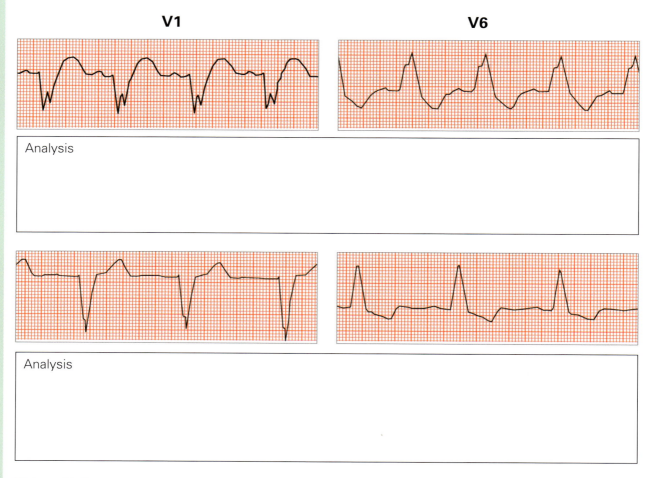

**Figure 11.5**

Chapter 12

# Chamber enlargement

When the heart has to face a chronic increase in pressure, either because of its inability to expel adequate amounts of blood from the left ventricle (increased preload) or because of resistance against expelling its contents (increased afterload), the muscular walls of the heart chambers thicken. This is known as **hypertrophy**.

## Left ventricular hypertrophy

An increase in the size of the left ventricle is called left ventricular hypertrophy. When the wall of the left ventricle increases in thickness, the heights of the QRS complexes increase. This is known as tall voltage. Tall voltage is usually present in Leads I, aVL, V5 and V6, as these are the leads that are recorded over the side of the left ventricle. Tall voltage will be recorded in the form of tall R waves (see fig 12.1).

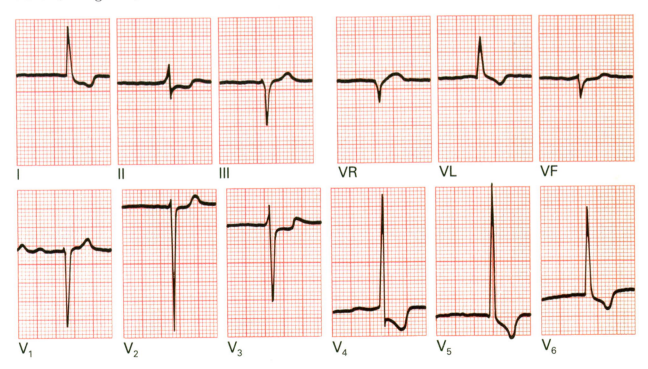

**Figure 12.1:** *Left ventricular hypertrophy.*

Several efforts have been made to lay down criteria on an ECG for the diagnosis of left ventricular hypertrophy. However, they have all been unreliable, as many other factors (including age and thickness of the chest wall) contribute to tall voltage. The ECG alone should not be used to make a diagnosis of hypertrophy. Instead, the practitioner should be encouraged to investigate the possibility further – ideally by **echocardiogram**.

The ancient but much-quoted criterion for left ventricular hypertrophy (proposed by Sokolow and Lyon, 1949), simply adds the depth of the S wave in V1 to the height of the R wave in either V5 or V6 (whichever is taller). If the sum is greater than 35 mm, left ventricular hypertrophy is suspected.

ST depression and T wave inversion are often present owing to repolarisation changes, in the left chest leads. This is sometimes referred to as a *strain* pattern. Its mechanics are not understood at present. However, myocardial ischaemia is a probable factor contributing to the pattern.

Left axis deviation may also be present because of the increased voltage over the left side of the heart.

## Right ventricular hypertrophy

An increase in the thickness of the walls of the right ventricle is called *right ventricular hypertrophy*. In the normal heart, the left ventricle is about three times as thick as the right. If the right ventricle is thinner than the left ventricle, hypertrophy of the right ventricle may go unnoticed on the ECG. If hypertrophy becomes severe, the right ventricular leads (V1 and V2) will increase their R wave voltages.

A criterion for recognition of right ventricle hypertrophy on an ECG has been suggested by Davis (1985):

● R wave is greater than or equal to S wave in V1
   *Or*
● R wave in V1 + S wave in V6 is greater than or equal to 10 mm

Once again, findings should be confirmed on echocardiogram.

Repolarisation changes are often present in the right ventricular leads, in the forms of ST depression and T wave inversion.

Right axis deviation may also be present.

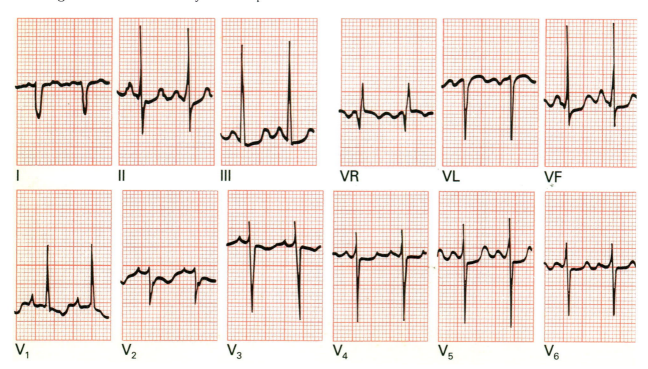

**Figure 12.2:** *Right ventricular hypertrophy.*

## Left atrial hypertrophy

An increase in the thickness of the left atrial wall is known as *left atrial hypertrophy*. This occurs frequently in left ventricular enlargement, although it can also occur alone. The *P wave is often widened* because of the increased time that it takes the impulse to travel over the thickened atrial wall. The P wave is notched, like an m shape (see fig 12.3). This is known as *P-mitrale*. In some leads (typically V1) *the P wave becomes negative*.

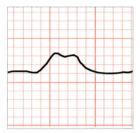

**Figure12.3:** *P-mitrale.*

## Right atrial hypertrophy

An increase in the thickness of the right atrium is known as *right atrial hypertrophy*. If the right atrium is hypertrophied there will be an *increase in the height of the P wave* (2.5 mm or more). This is seen most clearly in Lead II, and is due to the increase in the number of impulse directions travelling directly towards Lead II. The *P wave also looks peaked* (see fig 12.4). This is known as *P-pulmonale*. The width of the P wave is normal.

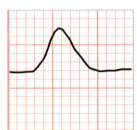

**Figure 12.4:** *P-pulmonale.*

## Activity 12.2: Atrial enlargement

*Approximate time required to complete this activity: 5 minutes*
*Answers are provided on p. 94.*

Fill the gaps in the following passage.

Atrial enlargement is shown on the ECG by changes to the _____ wave. Notably, the changes will

affect the _____ and the _____ of the wave.

When the right atrium is enlarged, the P wave is often > _____ mm in height and is _____

in appearance. This is sometimes referred to as P- _____.

When the left atrium is enlarged, the P wave is often _____, and has the appearance of an _____

shape. This is sometimes referred to as P-_____ .

Activities 12

# Chapter 13

# A systematic approach to ECG interpretation

Accurate ECG interpretation requires experience. However, applying a simple, systematic approach should enable you to interpret most of the ECGs you encounter. It may also provide diagnostic information and help direct appropriate treatment.

Here is a simple summary of the systematic approach to ECG interpretation as used in this book. This should help you to identify abnormalities on a 12 lead ECG quickly and easily.

## Rhythm strip

- Rate? (Count the number of QRS complexes in 30 squares x 10)
- Rhythm? (Regular/irregular?)
- Atrial activity?
- Ventricular activity?
- Relationship between atrial and ventricular activity. If abnormal, consider heart block.
- Measure:
  P wave ( < 2 small squares)
  PR interval ( < 5 small squares)      If longer, suspect first degree heart block
  QRS complex ( < 3 small squares)   If wide = ventricular rhythm
                                                                    If narrow/normal = atrial rhythm

## Heart block?

- First degree AV heart block (Prolonged PR interval)
- Second degree AV heart block
  Wenkebach (Gradual increased prolongation of PR interval)
  Mobitz II (Dropped beats but constant PR interval)
- Third degree AV heart block (Complete)
  No association with P and QRS waves
- Name or describe the trace

## 12 lead ECG

- Polarity of limb leads (aVR should be negative, all others should be positive)
- Axis deviation (I and aVF)
  Left  (leaving)

Right (reaching)
Extreme (both negative)

- Choose the smallest equiphasic complex in the limb leads.
- Find the corresponding lead. Move 90 degrees towards the appropriate section.
- R wave progression (V1–V6)   Good or poor?
  Is there:
  - Ischaemia  (ST depression, T wave inversion, T wave flattening)
  - Injury  (ST elevation)
  - Or necrosis? (Q waves, indicate full thickness MI)
- Which leads are affected?

### Myocardial infarction?

- Posterior MI
  Suspect if ST depression or tall R waves in V1 and V2
- Non ST elevation MI
  Non-resolving T wave inversion or ST depression and Troponin rise
- Diagnosis
  Which coronary vessels are affected?

### Bundle branch block

- Wide QRS complexes
- Look at V1 and V6
- Left bundle branch block (WILLIAM)
- Right bundle branch block (MARROW)

### Ventricular hypertrophy

- Left V4, V5, V6 high voltage
  R wave in V5 or V6 >25 mm
  R wave in V5 or V6 plus the S wave >35 mm
  R wave in V5 >20 mm
  Left axis deviation, ST depression, T inversion in V4–V6
  P-mitrale (P wave m-shaped)
- Right R wave >S in V1 >5 mm
  R wave in V1 plus the S wave in V5 or V6 >10 mm
  Right axis deviation, ST depression, T inversion in V1–V3
  P-pulmonale (P wave is peak-shaped)

# Answers to activities

## Activity 2.1

The ECG records electrical impulses as they pass through the specialised cells of the conducting system. As the electrical impulses pass across these cells, myocardial contraction occurs. Normally, all electrical impulses originate from the sino-atrial node in the right atrium. After spreading across the atria, the impulses then pass through the atrioventricular node and into the Bundle of His. The impulse spreads through the interventricular septum via the right and left bundle branches. Finally, the impulse conducts across the ventricular myocardium, causing contraction.

The ECG is made up of a number of parts, each of which relates to a different part of the conduction system. The first part of the normal ECG complex is the P wave. This represents the impulses that arise from the sino-atrial node and spread across the atria towards the atrioventricular node. As the impulse spreads across the ventricular myocardium, the ECG records a large wave called the QRS complex.

The spread of impulse across the atria and ventricles is often referred to as depolarisation. The total time that it takes for depolarisation to spread from the SA node to the ventricular myocardium is measured on the ECG as the PR interval. When the ventricles recover from depolarisation, the final part of the ECG complex is recorded. This is the T wave and represents repolarisation of the ventricles.

## Activity 3.1

### Scenario 1

| What is the rate? | ´40bpm |
|---|---|
| Is it regular or irregular? | Irregular |
| Is there atrial activity? (P waves) | No |
| Is there ventricular activity? (QRS complexes) | Yes |
| Are the QRS complexes broad or narrow? | Narrow |
| Is there a relationship between the atrial activity and the ventricular activity? | NA – there are no P waves |
| Are the PR intervals normal? | NA – there are no P waves |
| Name/description? | Atrial fibrillation |

**Scenario 2**

| What is the rate? | 120bpm |
|---|---|
| Is it regular or irregular? | Regular |
| Is there atrial activity? (P waves) | Yes |
| Is there ventricular activity? (QRS complexes) | Yes |
| Are the QRS complexes broad or narrow? | Narrow |
| Is there a relationship between the atrial activity and the ventricular activity? | Yes |
| Are the PR intervals normal? | Yes |
| Name/description? | Sinus tachycardia |

## Activity 4.1

| | ECG 1 | ECG 2 | ECG 3 |
|---|---|---|---|
| Is there atrial activity? | Yes | Yes | Yes |
| Are the P waves regular? | Yes | Yes | Yes |
| Is the ventricular activity regular? | No | Yes | Yes |
| Is the PR interval constant or does it vary? | Constant before QRS complexes | Varies | Constant |
| If the PR interval is constant, is it normal? | Yes | N/A | No |
| Are there missed QRS complexes? | Yes | No | No |
| What is this heart block? | Second degree (Mobitz type II) | Complete Heart Block | First degree |

## Activity 4.2

**1 The ECG represents…**

  A The structure of the heart

  B Movement of electrical impulses through the heart ✔

  C Movement of blood through the heart

  D The state of the coronary arteries

**2 Electrical conduction of the heart's cells is also known as…**

  A Polarisation

  B Repolarisation

  C Depolarisation ✔

  D Defibrillation

**3 ECG paper speed should be...**

A  25cm/s

B  2.5mm/s

C  2.5m/s

D  25mm/s ✔

**4  1 millivolt is represented as...**

A  2 large squares on the vertical axis ✔

B  2 cm on the horizontal axis

C  1 large square on the horizontal axis

D  2 cm on the vertical axis

**5  One small square on the horizontal axis of the ECG paper is...**

A  0.4 seconds

B  0.04 seconds ✔

C  1 second

D  0.2 seconds

**6  One large square on the horizontal axis of the ECG paper is...**

A  0.04 seconds

B  1 second

C  0.2 seconds ✔

D  0.02 seconds

**7  Which of these will not cause artefact on an ECG?**

A  Patient movement

B  Electrical apparatus

C  Palpitations ✔

D  Poor electrode contact

**8  Lead V4 is positioned...**

A  In the fourth intercostal space on the right sternal border

B  In the fourth intercostal space on the left sternal border

C  In the fifth intercostal space on the midaxillary line

D  In the fifth intercostal space on the mid-clavicular line ✔

**9  The width of the QRS should be...**

A  < 0.12 seconds ✔

B  > 0.12 seconds

C  0.12–2.0 seconds

D  > 2 seconds

**10 An ECG is 'Sinus' if …**

    A  It has a QRS complex

    B  It has a P wave ✔

    C  It has a T wave

    D  The ventricular rate is regular

**11      Lead position**                                **Lead**

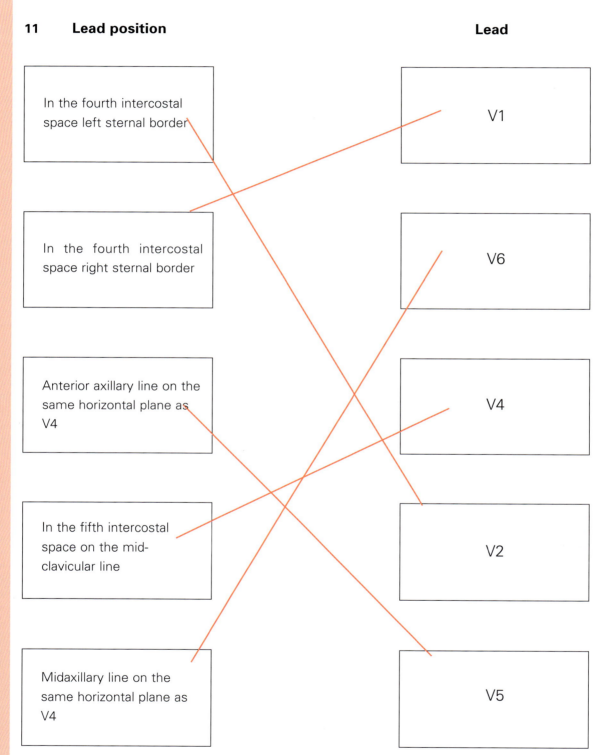

In the fourth intercostal space left sternal border

In the fourth intercostal space right sternal border

Anterior axillary line on the same horizontal plane as V4

In the fifth intercostal space on the mid-clavicular line

Midaxillary line on the same horizontal plane as V4

V1

V6

V4

V2

V5

**12**

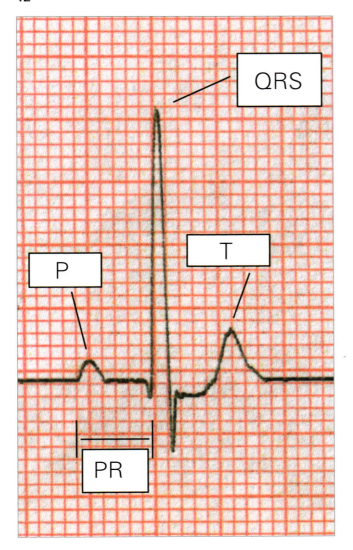

## Activity 5.1

**A** Ventricular tachycardia

**B** Atrial flutter

**C** Ventricular fibrillation

**D** Atrial fibrillation

**E** Supraventricular tachycardia

## Activity 6.1

**Figure 6.3a**: Ventricular (3rd complex)

**Figure 6.3b**: Atrial (complexes 2, 4 and 6)

**Figure 6.3c**: Ventricular (5th complex)

Answers

## Activity 7.1

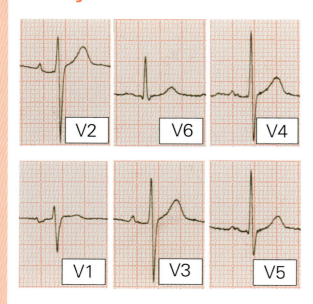

## Activity 8.1

### ECG 1

| Lead I is | + | (positive or negative). |
| Lead aVF | + | (positive or negative). |
| Therefore the axis is | normal | (left, right or normal). |

Lead __aVL__ is the smallest equiphasic lead. Lead ___II___ is 90 degrees to the most equiphasic lead. Therefore, the cardiac axis is __+60__ degrees.

### ECG 2

| Lead I is | + | (positive or negative). |
| Lead aVF | − | (positive or negative). |
| Therefore the axis is | left | (left, right or normal). |

Lead __aVR__ is the smallest equiphasic lead. Lead ___III___ is 90 degrees to the most equiphasic lead. Therefore, the cardiac axis is __-60__ degrees.

Answers

## Activity 9.1

| ECG lead | N for 'no' or Y for 'yes', as appropriate | | | | | |
|---|---|---|---|---|---|---|
| | Q waves? | ST elevation? | ST depression? | T wave inversion? | T wave flattening? | Likely cause/s (ischaemia, injury, necrosis) |
| I | N | N | Y | N | N | ischaemia |
| II | N | Y | N | N | N | injury |
| III | N | Y | N | N | N | injury |
| aVR | N | N | N | Y | N | lead not used to access these criteria |
| aVL | N | N | Y | N | N | ischaemia |
| aVF | N | Y | N | N | N | injury |
| V1 | N | N | N | Y | N | ischaemia |
| V2 | N | N | Y | N | N | ischaemia |
| V3 | N | N | Y | N | N | ischaemia |
| V4 | N | N | Y | N | N | ischaemia |
| V5 | N | N | Y | N | N | ischaemia |
| V6 | N | N | Y | N | N | ischaemia |

**NB:** The ischaemic changes seen in the chest leads are most likely to be reciprocal changes from the inferior ST elevations (II, III and aVF).

## Activity 10.1

**Myocardial region**

**ECG leads**

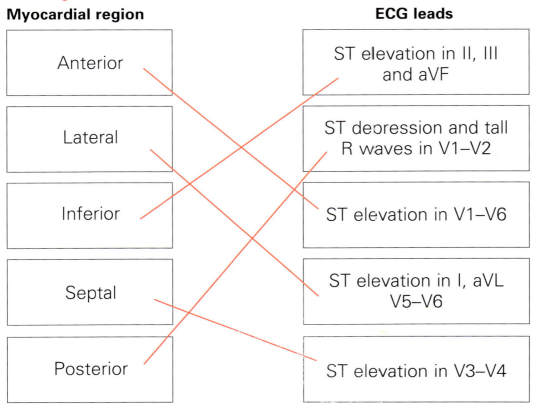

## Activity 10.2

**ECG 1:** Anterior Septal; ST elevations in Leads V1–V3

**ECG 2:** Inferior; ST elevation in Leads II, III, aVF.

## Activity 11.1

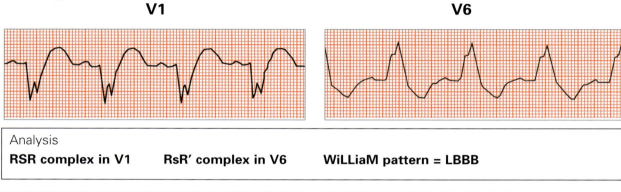

| V1 | V6 |
|---|---|

Analysis

**RSR complex in V1      RsR' complex in V6      WiLLiaM pattern = LBBB**

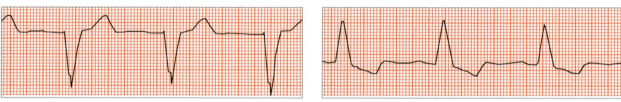

Analysis

**RsR complex in V1 (note the slight notch in the downstroke).**
**RS complex (very subtle notch in the downstroke) in V6.      WiLLiaM pattern= LBBB**

## Activity 12.1

Rate 200bpm

Regular

No obvious P waves

QRS present but narrow

Name: Narrow complex tachycardia or Supraventricular tachycardia (SVT)

Normal axis deviation +60 degrees

Ischaemic  changes  I II III aVL V2–V6

Deep S waves V1–V3 ?left ventricular enlargement

## Activity 12.2

Atrial enlargement is shown on the ECG by changes to the P wave. Notably, the changes will affect the height and the morphology (or shape) of the wave.

When the right atrium is enlarged, the P wave is often > 2.5 mm in height and is peaked in appearance. This is sometimes referred to as P-pulmonale.

When the left atrium is enlarged, the P wave is often notched and has the appearance of an M shape. This is sometimes referred to as P-mitrale.

# References

Adams, J.E., Bodor, G.S., Davila-Roma, V.G. et al. (1993). 'Cardiac troponin I: a marker with high specificity for cardiac injury' in *Circulation*, **88**, pp. 101–6.

Antman, E.M., Tanasijevic, M.J., Thompson, B. *et al.* (1996). 'Cardiac specific Troponin I levels to predict the risk of mortality of patients with acute coronary syndromes' in the *New England Journal of Medicine*, **335**, pp. 1342–9.

Bayley, R.H. (1944). 'Electrocardiographic changes (local ventricular ischaemia and injury) produced in the dog by temporary occlusion of a coronary artery, showing a new stage in the evolution of a myocardial infarction' in the *American Heart Journal*, **27**, p.164.

DANAMI-2 trial (2003). Anderson, H.R., Nielsen, T.T., Rasmussen, K., Thuesen, L., Kelbaek, P. et al. for the DANAMI -2 Investigators. 'A comparison of coronary angioplasty with fibrinolytic therapy in acute myocardial infarction' in the *New England Journal of Medicine*, **349**, pp. 733–42.

Davis, D. (1985). *How to Quickly and Accurately Master ECG Interpretation*, Philadelphia: J.B. Lippincott Company.

Department of Health (2000). 'The National Service Framework Document for Coronary Heart Disease'.

Fye, W.B. (1994). 'A history of the origin, evolution and impact of electrophysiology' in the *American Journal of Cardiology*, **73**, pp. 937–49.

Julian, D.G. and Cowan, J.C. (1992). *Cardiology*, 6th edn. London: Baillière Tindall.

Kourtesis, P. (1976). 'Incidence and significance of left anterior hemiblock complicating acute inferior myocardial infarction' in *Circulation*, **53**, p. 784.

Resuscitation Council UK (2005). *Advanced Life Support Manual*, 5th edn. London: The Resuscitation Council UK.

Rude, R.E., Poole, W.K., Muller J.E. *et al.* (1983). 'Electrocardiographic and clinical criteria for recognition of acute myocardial infarction based on analysis of 3,697 patients' in the *American Journal of Cardiology*, **52**, pp. 936–42.

Sokolow, M. and Lyon, T.P. (1949). 'The ventricular complex in left ventricular hypertrophy as obtained by unipolar precordial and limb leads' in the *American Heart Journal*, **37**, p. 161.

Springings, D., Chambers, J. and Jeffrey, A. (1995). *Acute Medicine*. Oxford: Blackwell Science Ltd.

**myocardium**  The middle (muscular) layer of the heart.

**occluded**  Blocked so that blood cannot flow.

**pericarditis**  Inflammation of the pericardium (the outermost layer of the heart).

**polarity**  Relating to the electrical poles (positive and negative) of the cardiac cell.

**primary angioplasty**  An invasive technique for opening up occluded blood vessels. The procedure is performed by introducing a catheter up through the femoral artery to the heart. This enables a balloon to be inflated in order to open up the artery (balloon angioplasty). Alternatively, a metal structure (stent) can be used to keep the artery open.

**pro-arrhythmic**  Putting the patient at risk of arrhythmias.

**R on T phenomenon**  This occurs when a ventricular ectopic falls so early that its R wave interrupts the T wave of the preceding complex, resulting in a high risk of ventricular tachycardia or fibrillation. The apex of the T wave is a vulnerable phase in the ventricular cycle. If stimulated by an ectopic, it may produce repeated ventricular responses, leading to life-threatening arrhythmias.

**repolarisation**  When a depolarised cell starts to return to its resting state.

**revascularisation**  A procedure to open up occluded blood vessels. This can be achieved by primary angioplasty or by thrombolysis.

**septum**  The wall of myocardium that lies between the atria and the ventricles.

**stent**  A stent is a tube placed in the coronary arteries to keep the arteries open while coronary artery disease is being treated. A stent is used in a procedure called percutaneous coronary intervention (PCI) or angioplasty.

**sternal notch**  A depression that is felt at the top of the sternal bone in the front, centre of the chest wall.

**tachyarrhythmia**  An abnormal heart rhythm that is faster than 120 beats per minute.

**tachycardia**  A heart rate that is faster than 100 beats per minute.

**thrombolysis**  The administration of a powerful drug to dissolve the clots that occlude the arteries.

**tricuspid valve**  The heart valve that lies between the right atrium and the right ventricle.

**troponin**  A small component of the myocardial cell that is released into the blood when myocardial injury occurs. Troponin is not normally present in the blood so measurement of troponin is a useful means of diagnosing myocardial infarction.

**vena cava**  The major veins that bring venous blood back to the heart. The superior vena cava brings blood from the upper body and the inferior vena cava brings blood from the lower body.

**ventricles**  The two larger heart chambers that eject the blood into the arteries. The right ventricle ejects blood into the pulmonary artery and the left ventricle ejects blood into the aorta.

# Index